T0259131

# INTERVENTIONAL CARDIOLOGY CLINICS

www.interventional.theclinics.com

*Editor-in-Chief*

MARVIN H. ENG

# Left Atrial Appendage Occlusion

April 2022 • Volume 11 • Number 2

*Editor*

MATTHEW J. DANIELS

**ELSEVIER**

1600 John F. Kennedy Boulevard • Suite 1800 • Philadelphia, Pennsylvania, 19103-2899

http://www.theclinics.com

**INTERVENTIONAL CARDIOLOGY CLINICS Volume 11, Number 2**
**April 2022 ISSN 2211-7458, ISBN-13: 978-0-323-89756-3**

Editor: Joanna Collett
Developmental Editor: Arlene B. Campos

© **2022 Elsevier Inc. All rights reserved.**

This periodical and the individual contributions contained in it are protected under copyright by Elsevier, and the following terms and conditions apply to their use:

**Photocopying**
Single photocopies of single articles may be made for personal use as allowed by national copyright laws. Permission of the Publisher and payment of a fee is required for all other photocopying, including multiple or systematic copying, copying for advertising or promotional purposes, resale, and all forms of document delivery. Special rates are available for educational institutions that wish to make photocopies for non-profit educational classroom use. For information on how to seek permission visit www.elsevier.com/permissions or call: (+44) 1865 843830 (UK)/(+1) 215 239 3804 (USA).

**Derivative Works**
Subscribers may reproduce tables of contents or prepare lists of articles including abstracts for internal circulation within their institutions. Permission of the Publisher is required for resale or distribution outside the institution. Permission of the Publisher is required for all other derivative works, including compilations and translations (please consult www.elsevier.com/permissions).

**Electronic Storage or Usage**
Permission of the Publisher is required to store or use electronically any material contained in this periodical, including any article or part of an article (please consult www.elsevier.com/permissions). Except as outlined above, no part of this publication may be reproduced, stored in a retrieval system or transmitted in any form or by any means, electronic, mechanical, photocopying, recording or otherwise, without prior written permission of the Publisher.

**Notice**
No responsibility is assumed by the Publisher for any injury and/or damage to persons or property as a matter of products liability, negligence or otherwise, or from any use or operation of any methods, products, instructions or ideas contained in the material herein. Because of rapid advances in the medical sciences, in particular, independent verification of diagnoses and drug dosages should be made.

Although all advertising material is expected to conform to ethical (medical) standards, inclusion in this publication does not constitute a guarantee or endorsement of the quality or value of such product or of the claims made of it by its manufacturer.

*Interventional Cardiology Clinics* (ISSN 2211-7458) is published quarterly by Elsevier Inc., 360 Park Avenue South, New York, NY 10010-1710. Months of issue are January, April, July, and October. Subscription prices are USD 209 per year for US individuals, USD 641 for US institutions, USD 100 per year for US students, USD 209 per year for Canadian individuals, USD 660 for Canadian institutions, USD 100 per year for Canadian students, USD 296 per year for international individuals, USD 660 for international institutions, and USD 150 per year for international students. To receive student/resident rate, orders must be accompanied by name of affiliated institution, date of term, and the *signature* of program/residency coordinator on institution letterhead. Orders will be billed at individual rate until proof of status is received. Foreign air speed delivery is included in all *Clinics* subscription prices. All prices are subject to change without notice. **POSTMASTER:** Send address changes to *Interventional Cardiology Clinics*, Elsevier Health Sciences Division, Subscription Customer Service, 3251 Riverport Lane, Maryland Heights, MO 63043. **Customer Service: Telephone: 1-800-654-2452** (U.S. and Canada); **1-314-447-8871** (outside U.S. and Canada). **Fax: 1-314-447-8029. E-mail: journalscustomerservice-usa@elsevier. com (for print support); journalsonlinesupport-usa@elsevier.com (for online support).**

*Reprints.* For copies of 100 or more of articles in this publication, please contact the Commercial Reprints Department, Elsevier Inc., 360 Park Avenue South, New York, NY 10010-1710. Tel.: 212-633-3874; Fax: 212-633-3820; E-mail: reprints@elsevier.com.

# CONTRIBUTORS

**EDITOR-IN-CHIEF**

**MARVIN H. ENG, MD**
Structural Heart Program Medical Director,
Structural Heart Disease Fellowship Director,
Director of Cardiovascular Quality, Banner
University Medical Center, Phoenix, Arizona,
USA

**EDITOR**

**MATTHEW J. DANIELS, BSc, MA, MB,
BChir, PhD, MRCP, FSCAI**
Senior Lecturer and Honorary Consultant
Cardiologist, Manchester Heart Centre,
Manchester Royal Infirmary, Manchester
University NHS Foundation Trust, Division of
Cardiovascular Sciences, Manchester
Academic Health Sciences Centre, Division of
Cell Matrix Biology and Regenerative
Medicine, University of Manchester,
Manchester, United Kingdom

**AUTHORS**

**MESFER ALFADHEL, MD**
Division of Cardiology, Vancouver General
Hospital, University of British Columbia,
Vancouver, British Columbia, Canada

**MOHAMAD ALKHOULI, MD**
Department of Cardiology, Professor of
Medicine, Mayo Clinic School of Medicine,
Rochester, Minnesota, USA

**DABIT ARZAMENDI, MD, PhD**
Department of Cardiology, Hospital de la Santa
Creu I Sant Pau, Centro de Investigación
Biomédica en Red de Enfermedades
Cardiovasculares (CIBERCV), Barcelona, Spain

**LLUIS ASMARATS, MD, PhD**
Department of Cardiology, Hospital de la
Santa Creu I Sant Pau, Barcelona, Spain

**OSCAR CAMARA, PhD**
Department of Information and
Communication Technologies, Universitat
Pompeu Fabra, Barcelona, Spain

**ALBERTO CRESTI, MD**
Cardiology Department, Misericordia
Hospital, Azienda Sanitaria Toscana SudEst,
Grosseto, Italy

**MATTHEW J. DANIELS, BSc, MA, MB,
BChir, PhD, MRCP, FSCAI**
Senior Lecturer and Honorary Consultant
Cardiologist, Manchester Heart Centre,
Manchester Royal Infirmary, Manchester
University NHS Foundation Trust, Division of
Cardiovascular Sciences, Manchester
Academic Health Sciences Centre, Division of
Cell Matrix Biology and Regenerative
Medicine, University of Manchester,
Manchester, United Kingdom

**OLE DE BACKER, MD, PhD, FESC**
The Heart Centre, Rigshospitalet,
Copenhagen University Hospital,
Copenhagen, Denmark

**TOM DE POTTER, MD**
Cardiovascular Center, Onze-Lieve-
Vrouwziekenhuis Hospital, Aalst, Belgium

**JASNEET DEVGUN, DO**
Division of Cardiology, Henry Ford Health
System, Detroit, Michigan, USA

**WERN YEW DING, MRCP**
Liverpool Centre for Cardiovascular Science,
University of Liverpool and Liverpool Heart
and Chest Hospital, Liverpool, United
Kingdom

**DAVIDE FABBRICATORE, MD**
Cardiovascular Center, Onze-Lieve-
Vrouwziekenhuis Hospital, Aalst, Belgium

**DHIRAJ GUPTA, MD**
Liverpool Centre for Cardiovascular Science,
University of Liverpool and Liverpool Heart
and Chest Hospital, Liverpool, United
Kingdom

**MAHMUT EDIP GUROL, MD, MSc**
Department of Neurology, Massachusetts
General Hospital, Harvard Medical School,
Boston, Massachusetts, USA

**THORSTEN HANKE, MD**
Professor of Surgery, Clinic for Cardiac
Surgery, Department of Cardiovascular
Surgery, ASKLEPIOS Klinikum Harburg,
Abteilung Herzchirurgie, Hamburg, Germany

**RANDALL J. LEE, MD, PhD**
Professor of Medicine, Cardiac
Electrophysiology, University of California,
San Francisco, San Francisco, California, USA

**GREGORY Y.H. LIP, MD**
Liverpool Centre for Cardiovascular Science,
University of Liverpool and Liverpool Heart
and Chest Hospital, Liverpool, United
Kingdom; Aalborg Thrombosis Research Unit,
Department of Clinical Medicine, Aalborg
University, Aalborg, Denmark

**CAMERON MCALISTER, MD**
Division of Cardiology, Vancouver General
Hospital, University of British Columbia,
Vancouver, British Columbia, Canada

**GWILYM M. MORRIS, BMBCh, PhD**
Division of Cardiovascular Sciences, The
University of Manchester, Manchester Heart
Centre, Manchester University NHS Foundation
Trust, Manchester, United Kingdom

**THOMAS NESTELBERGER, MD**
Division of Cardiology, Vancouver General
Hospital, University of British Columbia,
Vancouver, British Columbia, Canada;
Cardiovascular Research Institute Basel (CRIB),
Department of Cardiology, University Hospital
Basel, University of Basel, Basel, Switzerland

**JENS ERIK NIELSEN-KUDSK, MD, DMSc**
Department of Cardiology, Aarhus University
Hospital, Aarhus, Denmark

**ADRIAN PARRY-JONES, MD**
Division of Cardiovascular Sciences, University
of Manchester, Geoffrey Jefferson Brain

Research Centre, Manchester Academic
Health Science Centre, Northern Care Alliance
and University of Manchester, Manchester,
United Kingdom; Manchester Centre for
Clinical Neurosciences, Northern Care
Alliance NHS Group, Stott Lane, Salford,
United Kingdom

**TAMRA RANASINGHE, MD**
Department of Neurology, Wake Forest
School of Medicine, Winston-Salem, North
Carolina, USA

**LARS SØNDERGAARD, MD, DMSc**
The Heart Centre, Rigshospitalet,
Copenhagen University Hospital,
Copenhagen, Denmark

**KARAN SARAF, MBChB, MRCP**
Division of Cardiovascular Sciences, The
University of Manchester, Manchester Heart
Centre, Manchester University NHS
Foundation Trust, Manchester, United
Kingdom

**JACQUELINE SAW, MD**
Division of Cardiology, Vancouver General
Hospital, Clinical Professor, University of
British Columbia, Vancouver, British
Columbia, Canada; Interventional Cardiology,
Vancouver General Hospital, Basel, British
Columbia, Canada

**KOLJA SIEVERT, MD**
CardioVascular Center Frankfurt, St. Catherine
Hospital, Frankfurt, Germany

**APOSTOLOS TZIKAS, MD, PhD**
European Interbalkan Medical Centre and
AHEPA University Hospital, Thessaloniki,
Greece

**DEE DEE WANG, MD**
Division of Cardiology, Henry Ford Health
System, Detroit, Michigan, USA

**IVAN WONG, MD**
The Heart Centre, Rigshospitalet,
Copenhagen University Hospital,
Copenhagen, Denmark

# CONTENTS

A comprehensive evaluation is necessary to identify the etiologic factors in order to select optimal stroke-prevention measures. Atrial fibrillation is one of the most important stroke causes. Although anticoagulant therapy is the treatment of choice for patients with nonvalvular atrial fibrillation, it should not be considered uniformly to treat all patients given the high mortality associated with anticoagulant-related hemorrhages. The authors propose a risk-stratified individualized approach for stroke prevention in patients with nonvalvular atrial fibrillation by considering nonpharmacologic approaches for patients at high hemorrhage risk or otherwise unsuitable for lifelong anticoagulation.

 Video content accompanies this article at http://www.interventional.theclinics.com

Although the left atrial appendage (LAA) seems useless, it has several critical functions that are not fully known yet, such as the causes for being the main origin of cardioembolic stroke. Difficulties arise due to the extreme range of LAA morphologic variability, making the definition of normality challenging and hampering the stratification of thrombotic risk. Furthermore, obtaining quantitative metrics of its anatomy and function from patient data is not straightforward. A multimodality imaging approach, using advanced computational tools for their analysis, allows a complete characterization of the LAA to individualize medical decisions related to left atrial thrombosis patients.

Left atrial appendage (LAA) occlusion is emerging as a viable alternative to oral anticoagulation in high-risk patients with atrial fibrillation. However, there remains limited evidence for this approach, especially in certain subgroups, and therefore patient selection is an important aspect of treatment. Here, the authors present arguments for LAA occlusion as either a last resort versus patient choice by evaluating contemporary studies on this topic and discuss practical steps in the approach of patients who may be suitable for LAA occlusion. Overall, an individualized and multidisciplinary team approach should be adopted in patients who are being considered for LAA occlusion.

In the wake of rapid advancement in cardiovascular procedural technologies, physician-led preprocedural planning utilizing multi-modality imaging training is increasingly recognized as invaluable for procedural accuracy. Left atrial appendage occlusion (LAAO) is one such procedure in which complications such as device leak, cardiac injury, and device embolization can be decreased substantially with incorporation of physician driven imaging and digital tools. We discuss the benefits of cardiac CT and 3D printing in preprocedural planning for the Heart Team, as well as novel applications by physicians of intraprocedural 3D angiography and dynamic fusion imaging. Furthermore, incorporation of computational modeling and artificial intelligence (AI) may yield promise. For optimal patient-centric procedural success, we advocate for standardized preprocedural imaging planning by physicians within the Heart Team as an essential part of LAAO.

Left atrial appendage closure (LAAC) has become a commonly used alternative to anticoagulation for stroke prevention in patients with atrial fibrillation. There is a growing interest in adopting a minimally invasive procedural approach using intracardiac echocardiography (ICE) and moderate sedation. In this article, we review the rational for and the data supporting ICE-guided LAAC and discuss the pros and cons of this approach.

Routine postprocedural imaging with transesophageal echocardiography or cardiac computed tomography angiography is the most commonly used imaging modality for follow-up surveillance usually performed 1 to 6 months after the procedure. Imaging enables recognition of well-suited and sealed devices in the left atrial appendage as well as of potential harmful complications such as peri-device leaks, device-related thrombus, and device embolization, which may lead to further surveillance observation with recurrent imaging, reinitiation of oral anticoagulants, or additional interventional procedures.

This review summarizes the evidence for left atrial appendage closure (LAAC) as an alternative to oral anticoagulation (OAC) for stroke prevention in atrial fibrillation. LAAC reduces hemorrhagic stroke and mortality versus warfarin, but is inferior for ischemic stroke reduction based on randomized data. Whilst a feasible treatment in OAC-ineligible patients, questions remain over procedural safety, and the improvement in complications observed in nonrandomized registries is uncorroborated by contemporary randomized trials. Management of device-related thrombus and peridevice leak remain unclear, and robust randomized data versus direct OACs are required before recommendations can be made for widespread adoption in OAC-eligible populations.

Endocardial left atrial appendage (LAA) occluders with a covering disc encompass a wide range of devices that share the common feature of a distal anchoring "body" and proximal covering "disc" design. This unique design feature has potential advantages in certain complex LAA anatomies and challenging clinical scenarios. The current review article summarizes the different features of established and novel devices, preprocedural imaging updates, intraprocedural technical considerations, and postprocedural follow-up issues specific to this category of LAA occluders.

Left atrial appendage closure aims to eliminate the stasis component of Virchow triad by eliminating a cul-de-sac that favors thrombosis, particularly when atrial contractility becomes inefficient, such as in atrial fibrillation. Left atrial appendage closure devices have a common objective of sealing the appendage completely, with device stability and avoidance of device thrombosis. Two main device designs have been used to perform left atrial appendage closure: those that use a pacifier design (lobe + disk) and those that use a plug (single lobe) design. This review highlights the potential features and benefits of the single-lobe devices.

Left atrial appendage (LAA) epicardial exclusion has been associated with addressing 2 potential deleterious consequences attributed to the LAA, namely, thrombus formation and an arrhythmogenic contributor in advanced forms of atrial fibrillation. With more than 60 years of history, the surgical exclusion of the LAA has been firmly established. Numerous approaches have been used for surgical LAA exclusion including surgical resections, suture ligation, cutting and non-cutting staples, and surgical clips. Additionally, a percutaneous epicardial LAA ligation approach has been developed. A discussion of the various epicardial LAA exclusion approaches and their efficacy will be discussed, along with the salient beneficial affects on LAA thrombus formation, LAA electrical isolation and neuroendocrine homeostasis.

Early experience with percutaneous LAA closure documented complication rates of ~10%, with failure to implant devices in ~10% of patients. These numbers are unrecognizable in contemporary practice due to the iterative changes made largely in the last 10 years. Here we look forward to ask what might change, and when, to bring percutaneous LAA closure out of the niche early adopter centers into routine use. We consider the opportunity to incorporate different technologies into LAAc devices in the context of managing patient with atrial fibrillation. Finally, we consider how to make the procedure safer and more effective.

# LEFT ATRIAL APPENDAGE OCCLUSION

**RELATED SERIES**

*Cardiology Clinics*
*Heart Failure Clinics*
*Cardiac Electrophysiology Clinics*

**THE CLINICS ARE NOW AVAILABLE ONLINE!**

Access your subscription at:
**www.theclinics.com**

# FOREWORD

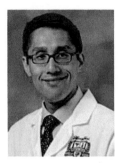

Marvin H. Eng, MD
*Consulting Editor*

This issue of Interventional Cardiology Clinics critically evaluates left atrial appendage occlusion (LAAO). The procedure is ubiquitous globally and several permutation of LAAO devices are currently under clinical development. The first generation WATCHMAN occluder is one of the most scrutinized devices to be approved by the United States Food and Drug Agency (FDA). The rigors of its testing may be testament of the controversy LAAO. In essence, LAAO is a prophylactic procedure, it preemptively seals the left atrial appendage in patients who cannot tolerate oral anticoagulation to prevent future thromboembolic events. To meet the burden of safety expected for prophylactic procedures, the complication rates must very low to justify the resources and risk of LAAO. In light of these facets of LAAO, this timely review will examine the fundamental aspects of LAAO to better prepare interested clinicians in providing the therapy.

Although LAAO superficially appears simple, more careful study of subject reveals several nuanced facets of the procedure that deserve attention. Debate on whether LAAO should be the default or secondary strategy in thromboembolic prevention in atrial fibrillation or secondary. Understanding left atrial appendage anatomy and its implications for LAAO is the basis for device design and procedural success. Imaging is key across the spectrum of structural procedures, LAAO included. Value of pre- and post-implant imaging is discussed. Advantages, limitations, and evidence base for different occlude device designs are explored in detail. Short and long-term projection of the LAAO field is provided. By posing open questions and providing in-depth analysis of contemporary literature, the authors challenge readership to imagining LAAO's future.

This latest issue of Interventional Cardiology Clinics reflects the multidisciplinary expertise required to advance the field of LAAO. We congratulate Dr. Matthew Daniels on assembling a comprehensive issue that concentrates the essential knowledge germane to advancing the field of LAAO.

Marvin H. Eng, MD
Banner University Medical Center
1111 East McDowell Road
Phoenix, AZ 85006, USA

*E-mail address:*
engm@email.arizona.edu

Intervent Cardiol Clin 11 (2022) ix
https://doi.org/10.1016/j.iccl.2022.02.001
2211-7458/22/© 2022 Published by Elsevier Inc.

# PREFACE

## Left Atrial Appendage Occlusion in 2022: Nearing Prime Time?

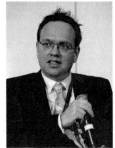

Matthew J. Daniels, BSc, MA, MB, BChir, PhD, MRCP,
FSCAI
*Editor*

Atrial fibrillation (AF) is common, and driven by rates of obesity and aging, is increasing. Consumer electronic devices, with capabilities to identify AF, bring an asymptomatic patient population to medical attention.

The security with which a diagnosis of AF can be made contrasts sharply with the certainties to treat it. A simple electrocardiogram is all that is required for diagnosis; thereafter things become taxing, as many aspects of AF management are unsatisfactory.

Classification is based crudely on how long it lasts in the patient, rather than subdivisions by causal aetiology, or anatomic/electrical subtypes. This lack of structure makes homogenous treatment paradigms inevitable.

Efforts to reduce the burden of AF pharmacologically, or invasively by elective catheter ablation, produce transient suppression in most cases. With no highly effective mechanism to turn back the tide of AF at the population level, incident diagnoses and treatment relapses outnumber the population gaining temporary cessation of disease progression. The consequences of AF (and their associated treatments) become the dominant health care burdens.

One consequence of AF is the risk of cardioembolic stroke. On a population level, we can estimate stroke risk, but on a patient level, we cannot define this with any certainty.

We can identify AF patients who are at low risk of stroke, the CHA$_2$DS$_2$-VASc zero group; yet low risk does not mean no risk. The annual risk of stroke is only lower than the risks of trying to prevent it by any means currently available. A significant proportion of strokes occurs in a group relatively unprotected in current guidelines. The best we can offer is to reclassify patients as high risk following stroke. A stroke prediction tool that works after the event, but not before it, is not a prediction tool. Perhaps we can do better, but the tools do not exist at present.

A higher-risk patient cohort that benefits from blood thinners, like warfarin, or the direct oral anticoagulants can be identified, the CHA$_2$DS$_2$-VASc 2+ cohort. Here, patients trade significant reductions in embolic stroke for a measureable, but overall smaller, increase in bleeding, yielding a net benefit overall. However, many patients, approximately 100,000 a year in the United States alone, have major bleeding events on these medications. Therefore, "net benefit" offers little to patients harmed, rather than helped, by their treatment.

Since many anticoagulant strategies prevent stroke in AF patients, a thrombotic mechanism connecting the electrical abnormality of the heart with the remote clinical consequence in the brain seems certain. However, the simple observation that there are more left atrial appendage (LAA)

Intervent Cardiol Clin 11 (2022) xi–xii
https://doi.org/10.1016/j.iccl.2022.01.002
2211-7458/22/© 2022 Published by Elsevier Inc.

thrombi in the AF patient cohort than there are patients experiencing embolic stroke demonstrates that intracardiac clot formation, and clot resolution (within the heart or the body), is a dynamic process. We know little of the factors tipping the balance toward clot formation, or resolution, which must change on a daily basis. Even simple parameters that we can measure are not easy to understand. Rapid flow within the appendage appears to prevent clot formation, but slow flow does not always cause it, for example.

The rules governing intracardiac clot formation in AF are complex. We know that we fail every low-risk patient admitted with embolic stroke who was falsely reassured that they didn't need to take an oral anticoagulant. We know that adverse bleeding events have the potential to be both life-threatening and terrifying for patients and their families. Just like stroke in the apparently low-risk patient, we are often wise after adverse bleeding events rather than before. Faced with these observations, it is no wonder that other avenues are being explored to try and alter the natural history of stroke associated with a common and simple-to-detect arrhythmia like AF.

The idea of a mechanical prophylactic intervention to prevent a future stroke is appealing. The LAA is a discrete, and effectively redundant, anatomic entity that is almost exclusively the site of intracardiac thrombus in AF. Hence, the notion of LAA exclusion by surgical or transcatheter means is gathering momentum as an alternative to systemic anticoagulation, which confers an inherent bleeding risk, in addition to the vulnerabilities of daily medication compliance, which limits efficacy.

Clearly, if the spectrum of possible interventions for the LAA could be delivered with zero risk, and complete success, there would be no need for this series of articles but at the time of writing this is a field that has not yet gotten close enough to the accepted hurdles for safety and efficacy to persuade the guideline writers to endorse such a position.

Here, some of the world's leading experts in this field produce a themed series of reviews that start with apparently simple questions relevant to clinical practice. These are developed reflecting the current state-of-the-art knowledge at the intersection between stroke and bleeding risk management in AF patients. Where relevant, I have asked authors to make binary decisions, which I accept may artificially polarize some of the discussions and conclusions reached, but it is hoped presents a clear narrative and conclusion for the reader to follow. As with any viewpoint, or perspective, different conclusions can be reached from the same starting point, so if you read something that you disagree with, please bring it up with your favorite meeting organizers and ask them to take it on as a debate topic!

Matthew J. Daniels, BSc, MA, MB, BChir, PhD, MRCP, FSCAI
Institute of Cardiovascular Sciences
Core Technology Facility
University of Manchester
Room 3.20, 46 Grafton Street
Manchester, M13 9NT, UK

*E-mail address:*
matthew.daniels@manchester.ac.uk

# Are Ischemic Strokes the Same? The Special Case Argument of Atrial Fibrillation

Tamra Ranasinghe, MD[a],
Mahmut Edip Gurol, MD, MSc[b],*

## KEYWORDS

- Stroke prevention • Atrial fibrillation • Ischemic stroke • Intracerebral hemorrhage
- Anticoagulation • Left atrial appendage closure

## KEY POINTS

- All ischemic strokes are not the same. A comprehensive etiologic evaluation is essential to understand the potential causes and risk factors for stroke.
- Atrial fibrillation is an important stroke cause, and it increases the risk of ischemic stroke and morbidity/mortality significantly. Although less common than ischemic strokes, anticoagulant-related brain hemorrhages have exceedingly high case-fatality and severe disability.
- Anticoagulants are the current treatment of choice for atrial fibrillation; however, comprehensive risk stratification is required before committing patients to lifelong anticoagulants because of their known hemorrhagic complications.
- Nonpharmacologic approaches, such as left atrial appendage closure, should be considered in patients with nonvalvular atrial fibrillation who are unable to tolerate long-term anticoagulation and/or who are at increased risk of hemorrhage.

## INTRODUCTION

Approximately 690,000 ischemic strokes (IS) occur each year in the United States, 185,000 of which are recurrent strokes.[1] The annual IS recurrence has shown a reduction from 8.7% in the 1960s to 5.0% in the 2000s probably owing to improved stroke-prevention therapies.[2] Although stroke mortality has decreased from the third leading cause of death in 1960s to the fifth leading cause of death in 2013,[3] it remains one of leading causes of serious long-term disability in the United States. This article addresses issues about different stroke causes that need to be understood by a large audience of nonneurologists in order to provide optimal preventive care, and the authors focus on particularities of IS-related to atrial fibrillation (AF) and its prevention.

## STROKE CAUSES AND THEIR IMPACT ON CHOICE OF STROKE-PREVENTION MEASURES

It is important to remember the fact that strokes are of 2 major types (ischemic vs hemorrhagic) and that, albeit less common, hemorrhagic strokes are 3 to 4 times more likely to be disabling or fatal when compared with IS.[4] Anticoagulant-related hemorrhagic strokes have a 1-month mortality of ~50%, making them one of the deadliest common medical emergencies known to humans.[4] Hence, it is imperative to be aware of concurrent risks while selecting lifelong anticoagulation versus

Study funding: M.E. Gurol: NIH funding (R01NS114526, NS083711).
[a] Department of Neurology, Wake Forest School of Medicine, 1 Medical Center Boulevard, Winston-Salem, NC 27157, USA; [b] Department of Neurology, Massachusetts General Hospital, Harvard Medical School, 175 Cambridge Street, Suite 300, Boston, MA 02114, USA
* Corresponding author.
*E-mail address:* edip@mail.harvard.edu

2211-7458/22/© 2021 Elsevier Inc. All rights reserved.

| Abbreviations | |
| --- | --- |
| AF | Atrial Fibrillation |
| cSVD | cerebral small vessel disease |
| ICM | insertable cardiac monitors |
| IS | Ischemic Stroke |

alternative nonpharmacologic approaches, such as left atrial appendage closure (LAAC) in the presence of AF. This issue is further discussed under the AF section later.

There are multiple IS causes other than AF that have different mechanisms and variable preventive treatments. Hence, there is no "one-size-fits-all" approach that can reduce stroke risk in patients with different causes. A comprehensive diagnostic evaluation is required to understand the potential causes along with an individualized treatment plan. There are a few general strategies that should be followed for secondary IS prevention in most situations. For secondary IS prevention, the recommended blood pressure goal is less than 130/80 mm Hg; low-density lipoprotein cholesterol goal is less than 70 mg/dL, and hemoglobin A1c goal is less than 7%.[5] These recommendations are mostly proven to decrease atherosclerotic IS risk, but they are used after all IS or transient ischemic attacks (TIA) unless there is a contraindication for a particular strategy.

There are 5 major etiologic categories for IS per TOAST (Trial of Org 10172 in Acute Stroke Treatment) classification: (1) cerebral small vessel disease (cSVD) -related lacunar infarction, (2) large artery atherosclerosis, (3) cardioembolism, (4) stroke of other determined cause, and (5) stroke of undetermined cause.[6] The authors briefly discuss the important aspects of these categories as they relate to prevention efforts before focusing on AF-related strokes.

Lacunar stroke is a subcortical IS measuring ≤1.5 cm in greatest diameter on brain computed tomography (CT) or MRI scan without evidence of concomitant cortical infarction. They are attributed to cSVD. History of hypertension, hyperlipidemia, and diabetes mellitus supports the clinical diagnosis. It is very important to remember that patients with cSVD are also at high risk of having an intracerebral hemorrhage (ICH) that is either fatal (∼50%) or severely disabling (∼30%) in the presence of anticoagulation. For this reason, providers should not escalate antithrombotics for cSVD-related strokes, unless there is another clear clinical indication for anticoagulant use. If cSVD-related lacunar infarct or infarcts or other evidence of cSVD, such as microbleeds, cortical superficial

siderosis, moderate-severe white matter disease, severe perivascular spaces, is present in a patient with AF, nonpharmacologic alternatives to lifelong anticoagulation such as LAAC should be considered. Recognition of these markers is important, and they have been discussed in great detail in recently published review articles.[7,8] Currently, the only proven long-term antithrombotic approach to decrease IS risk without disproportionately increasing hemorrhagic stroke risk in patients with cSVD is antiplatelet monotherapy, mainly aspirin.

Stroke caused by large artery atherosclerosis will demonstrate an infarction greater than 1.5 cm in diameter on brain CT or MRI scan in a vascular distribution of a major extracranial or intracranial artery with greater than 50% stenosis or occlusion of the corresponding proximal vessel on vascular imaging. Diagnostic studies should exclude potential sources of cardioembolism. Patients with stroke with symptomatic extracranial carotid artery atherosclerosis with 70% to 99% stenosis should be considered for either carotid endarterectomy or carotid artery stenting.[9,10] For patients with stroke with symptomatic extracranial carotid artery atherosclerosis with 50% to 69% stenosis, carotid endarterectomy is recommended depending on patient-specific factors, such as age, sex, and other comorbidities.[9] For patients with stroke with less than 50% extracranial carotid artery stenosis, revascularization procedures for secondary prevention are not recommended.[9] In patients with stroke and symptomatic intracranial atherosclerosis, addition of Clopidogrel 75 mg to aspirin for up to 90 days is reasonable to further reduce the early recurrent stroke risk.[11] When investigating for the cause of an IS or TIA, it is extremely important to evaluate for the presence of large vessel disease (extracranial and intracranial) using appropriate methods, as their management is different. Such diagnostic modalities include CT angiography of head and neck, magnetic resonance angiography of head and neck, carotid duplex of neck vessels, and transcranial Dopplers. The gold-standard diagnostic modality is the digital subtraction angiography, also referred to as the conventional cerebral angiography. Given the invasive nature of this investigation, it is obtained only in a select group of patients with IS requiring direct visualization of the head and neck vessel pathologic condition. Even when there is a potential obvious cause for an IS/TIA, vessel imaging of the head and neck is essential to complete the stroke workup. Failure to treat symptomatic large vessel pathologies appropriately has been implicated as a cause for oral anticoagulant (OAC) failure in patients with concomitant AF.

Cardioembolism category includes patients with arterial occlusions presumably owing to embolus arising from a cardiac source. Valvular heart disease, including infective endocarditis, left atrial thrombus, left ventricular thrombus, AF, cardiomyopathy, patent foramen ovale, and cardiac tumors, is a cause of cardioembolic stroke. Brain imaging would demonstrate cerebral cortical or cerebellar infarct, or brainstem or subcortical infarct greater than 1.5 cm in diameter without significant large vessel atherosclerosis on the head and neck vessel imaging. However, evidence of concomitant smaller strokes in more than one vascular territory suggests a cardioembolic/central cause. Long-term anticoagulant therapy should only be reserved for clearly identified stroke causes where clinical trials demonstrate robust evidence of efficacy, such as AF in patients suitable for anticoagulation or patients with mechanical heart valves. Anticoagulation should not be prescribed in a "uniform manner" for all cardioembolic strokes, as it did not prove to be beneficial in other situations, such as heart failure in the absence of AF or intracardiac thrombus.[12,13] As another example, in patients with infective endocarditis and stroke, treatment entails intravenous antibiotics and possible surgical valve replacement rather than anticoagulation therapy. Anticoagulant therapy is contraindicated in these patients, as it increases the risk of intracranial hemorrhage related to mycotic aneurysms and/or intracranial vessel wall involvement from septic emboli. AF is discussed in more detail in later sections.

Strokes of other determined cause include rare causes of IS, such as cervicocranial arterial dissections, hypercoagulable states, hematological disorders, nonatherosclerotic vasculopathies, and genetic disorders, to name a few. Lifelong anticoagulation is an established treatment for antiphospholipid antibody syndrome, but it is otherwise not proven to be of benefit for other categories.

Strokes of undetermined cause or cryptogenic strokes do not have a diagnosed stroke cause despite an adequate evaluation or could have 2 or more potential causes of stroke. Although a potentially misleading term, embolic stroke of undetermined source (ESUS) is used to describe nonlacunar cryptogenic strokes. They do not fit the lacunar stroke imaging criteria and appear embolic in nature, but an etiologic workup for IS does not yield a clear cause. All ESUS are cryptogenic strokes, but not all cryptogenic strokes are ESUS.

In 2 randomized controlled trials (RCT), treatment with Rivaroxaban or Dabigatran was not superior to aspirin in recurrent stroke prevention in patients with ESUS.[14,15] Furthermore, direct oral anticoagulation (DOAC) use was associated with higher bleeding risk, including up to 6.5 times higher risk of hemorrhagic stroke. Hence, use of DOAC should not be considered in patients with ESUS for stroke prevention. Long-term heart monitoring for patients with cryptogenic stroke with an external heart rhythm monitor, such as mobile cardiac outpatient telemetry or patch monitors and/or insertable cardiac monitors (ICM), is recommended to optimize detection of underlying paroxysmal AF. In an RCT of patients with cryptogenic stroke, AF was detected in 8.9% of patients with an ICM versus 1.4% of patients receiving conventional follow-up at 6 months, and the yield of ICM increased up to 8.8-fold over 3 years of follow-up.[16] Recently published data further demonstrated a 12.1% AF detection when patients with IS with a stroke cause diagnosed as large or small vessel disease were monitored over 12 months with an ICM.[17] The potential benefit of high-sensitivity long-term monitoring in this patient population is unknown, but it became clear that ICM provides very high yield in detection of AF in multiple different patient populations.

A major take-home message from this section is that an extensive stroke etiologic evaluation should be completed in all patients with IS and patients with TIA in order to select appropriate preventive strategies to minimize the risk of both recurrent ischemic and hemorrhagic strokes.

## THE SPECIAL CASE FOR ATRIAL FIBRILLATION AS A CAUSE OF ISCHEMIC STROKES AND PARTICULARITIES IN STROKE-PREVENTION STRATEGIES

AF is the most common arrhythmia in the adult population and is an important cause of cardioembolic stroke. AF affects ~6 million patients in the United States and is estimated to increase to 12 million by 2030.[18] AF is categorized as paroxysmal, persistent, or permanent depending on the time burden the patient experiences the arrhythmia. Higher AF burden is associated with a higher IS risk; however, there is no clearly established lower limit of AF time burden associated with embolism risk.[19]

Nonvalvular atrial fibrillation (NVAF) independently increases the IS risk by ~5-fold throughout all age groups[20]; however, the AF-related embolic risk depends on the population studied and the treatment plan. Data from phase III RCTs of DOACs clearly show the correlation between embolic risk and annual event rates. RE-LY (dabigatran)[21] and ARISTOTLE (apixaban)[22] showed annual IS risk around 1% in patients with NVAF who had mean CHADS2 of 2.1, whereas such annual IS risk was 1.35% in ROCKET AF (rivaroxaban),[23] a study that enrolled a higher embolic risk NVAF population (mean CHADS2 = 3.5). Finally, a recent observational prospective multicenter effort showed that patients with NVAF who had an IS despite using OAC, including DOACs, had a very high IS recurrence rate (8.9%) whether or not their anticoagulant was changed.[24]

An observational study demonstrated 18.2% prevalence of AF in hospitalized patients with IS, and the prevalence further increased to 40% in patients older than 85 years.[18] Multiple large studies across the globe have shown AF-related IS to be associated with worse short- and long-term mortality. An analysis of a registry from 7 European countries of 4462 patients with IS, the 3-month mortality of AF-related patients was 32.8% compared with 19.9% for patients with non-AF IS (P<.001).[25] A retrospective review of the National Inpatient Sample, which includes 1000 hospitals in 45 states in the United States from 2003 to 2014, observed 930,010 patients admitted with IS. Among these patients, 18.2% were diagnosed with AF. The in-hospital mortality in the matched cohorts with AF-related IS was 9.9% compared with 6.1% in patients with non-AF IS (P<.001).[18] In a Canadian prospective registry of 12,686 patients with IS, patients with AF-related stroke had higher rates of death at 1 month (22.3% vs 10.2%; P<.0001) and at 1 year (37.1% vs 19.5%; P<.0001) compared with the patients with non-AF stroke.[26] Similarly, a Japanese multicenter stroke registry of 15,831 patients demonstrated an 11.3%, 28-day mortality in patients with AF-related IS compared with 3.4% in the patients with non-AF IS (P<.0001).[27] Finally, a prospective analysis of a population-based study in North Dublin, Ireland followed 568 patients with IS over 5 years, and it observed a higher mortality, morbidity, stroke recurrence, and nursing home requirement in the AF-related stroke population.[28] A pooled analysis of 11 studies at 30 days and 4 studies at 1 year demonstrated patients with AF-related stroke are twice as likely to be dead at 30 days and at 1 year compared with non-AF strokes.[29]

Hemorrhagic strokes are associated with 3 to 4 times higher risk of mortality and severe disability when compared with IS. Anticoagulant-related hemorrhagic strokes have the highest fatality and disability among common medical emergencies.[4] A good understanding of these facts are very important to select appropriate preventive strategies in patients with AF. The current Food and Drug Administration (FDA)-approved stroke-prevention methods in patients with NVAF at high embolic risk as predicted by risk scores, such as CHA2DS2-VASc, are warfarin, DOACs, and LAAC.

In patients with stroke with AF, anticoagulation therapy is considered the treatment of choice for stroke prevention unless there is a contraindication for long-term anticoagulant use in which case LAAC needs to be considered. DOAC are recommended in preference to warfarin in patients with stroke with NVAF.[21–23,30] It is reasonable to initiate anticoagulation 2 to 14 days after index stroke in patients at low risk for hemorrhagic conversion.[31] Interestingly, the minimal duration of AF that engenders significant stroke risk and benefit of OAC beyond the bleeding risk remains unknown for primary stroke prevention.[5] It is safe to say that any duration of AF should trigger consideration for long-term anticoagulation or LAAC in patients with NVAF who had a stroke or TIA, as these patients represent a particularly high-risk category for embolism.

Reported annual rate of intracranial hemorrhage is 0.3% to 8% in patients on DOAC therapy depending on baseline risk: 46% to 52% are intracerebral; 17% to 45% are subdural; and 6% to 8% are subarachnoid hemorrhages.[21,23,32] The 30- to 90-day mortalities of 40% to 65% with anticoagulant-related ICH show the worst prognosis.

Lifelong full-dose anticoagulation therapy presents a special set of challenges: (1) it is associated with significant risks of both systematic hemorrhage and most importantly fatal or disabling brain hemorrhages; (2) nonadherence; (3) affordability; (4) over/underdosing; and (5) anticoagulant therapy failure. DOAC and warfarin failures, that is, recurrence of IS in patients with AF who were compliant on OAC, are commonly encountered in clinical practice.[31] There are no robust data or guidelines on how to manage these patients, causing a major challenge when considering whether to continue the same anticoagulant therapy or to switch to a different agent. The safety of prescribing warfarin/DOAC for patients with AF who sustained an ICH has been addressed in recent RCTs (So-START and APACHE-AF),[32,33] and these studies consistently showed higher brain bleeding rates when anticoagulant was resumed after an ICH (4- to 5-fold increased risk when compared with not starting anticoagulant).

Treatment of acute IS in patients with AF presents important challenges, as these are classically more severe strokes, and the use of full-dose systemic intravenous recombinant tissue plasminogen activator or even some endovascular recanalization treatments that require heparin during the procedure is either contraindicated or significantly risky in patients on effective OAC therapy.

Multiple lines of evidence suggest that the left atrial appendage is the main nidus of thrombus formation and thus embolism in AF.[34,35] The 5-year outcomes analysis after LAAC in PROTECT AF and PREVAIL trials, which randomized patients with NVAF to LAAC or warfarin in a 2:1 fashion, demonstrated LAAC with the WATCHMAN device provides secondary stroke prevention comparable to warfarin, while reducing major bleeding and mortality.[36] Given these trials and the FDA approval of now WATCHMAN FLX as well as AMPLATZER AMULET, LAAC is more widely used as a stroke-prevention approach that does not require lifelong OAC use. LAAC was included in the recently published 2021 secondary stroke-prevention guidelines for patients with NVAF who have contraindications for lifelong anticoagulation use but who can tolerate a short course of ~45 days.[5] A recent RCT demonstrated LAAC was noninferior to DOAC in preventing major AF-related cardiovascular, neurologic, and bleeding events, among patients at high risk for stroke and increased risk of bleeding.[37]

Currently, there are several LAAC devices implanted using transcatheter approaches approved in Europe and North America. The next-generation WATCHMAN FLX proved to have very low major procedural complication rates (0.5%) and 100% successful closure rates, leading to the FDA approval of this new device.[38] The AMPLATZER AMULET device was compared with first-generation WATCHMAN, and it proved noninferior for safety and efficacy endpoints, leading to its approval in the United States.[39] These nonpharmacologic approaches and technologies provide additional options for stroke prevention in NVAF, minimizing the risk of bleeding that comes with long-term anticoagulant therapy, and providing high rates of anatomic closure with a low incidence of adverse events.[40] Physicians should perform a stratification of ICH and other hemorrhagic risk based on not only clinical risk factors but also imaging findings, such as microbleeds, cortical superficial siderosis, and leukoaraiosis among others, and discuss LAAC as an alternative for patients who have either high ICH risk, for patients who have other hemorrhage risk, and indeed, in patients unsuitable for lifelong anticoagulation.[4,7,8] For a comprehensive risk stratification of OAC use in patients with AF without a prior history of stroke/TIA, a special consideration can be made on a case-by-case basis to obtain an MRI brain scan to screen for high-bleeding-risk imaging findings.

## SUMMARY

All IS are not the same; hence, understanding the cause of IS is of paramount importance when selecting effective preventive approaches. There is no "one-size-fits-all" treatment especially when it comes to antithrombotic approaches. Anticoagulant therapy for IS prevention should be considered judiciously in patients with NVAF who do have high hemorrhagic risk. The authors emphasize the importance of diagnosing AF appropriately, stratifying ischemic and hemorrhagic stroke risk to determine an individualized preventive approach for NVAF-related IS, that is, lifelong OAC therapy versus LAAC, in high-bleeding-risk patients and other patients unsuitable for long-term OAC use.

## CLINICS CARE POINTS

- Anticoagulant therapy is not recommended for patients with embolic strokes of unknown source.

- Anticoagulant-related hemorrhagic strokes have a very high fatality (50%–70%) and disability rate.

- Brain MRI markers of lacunar infarctions, microbleeds, cortical superficial siderosis, moderate-severe white matter disease, and severe perivascular spaces are associated with increased risk of intracranial hemorrhage.

- Left atrial appendage is the main nidus of thrombus formation in patients with atrial fibrillation.

- Randomized controlled studies of patients with nonvalvular atrial fibrillation treated with left atrial appendage closure have demonstrated noninferiority in stroke prevention while reducing major bleeding in comparison to oral anticoagulants.

- Nonpharmacologic approaches for stroke prevention in patients with nonvalvular atrial fibrillation should be considered in patients at high hemorrhage risk as well as in patients who cannot tolerate long-term anticoagulant use.
- There are 2 left atrial appendage closure devices (WATCHMAN FLX and AMPLATZER AMULET) currently approved by the Food and Drug Administration for stroke prevention in the United States.

## DISCLOSURE

T. Ranasinghe: no disclosures. M.E. Gurol: Neurocardiology section editor, American Heart Association *Stroke* journal; Chair, WSO Task Force on Cerebral Small Vessel Diseases and Vascular Cognitive Impairment; Member, WSO Brain & Heart Task Force; M.E.G.'s hospital received research funding from AVID, Pfizer, and Boston Scientific Corporation.

## REFERENCES

1. Virani SS, Alonso A, Benjamin EJ, et al. on behalf of the American Heart Association Council on Epidemiology and Prevention Statistics Committee and Stroke Statistics Subcommittee. Heart disease and stroke statistics–2020 update: a report from the American Heart Association. Circulation 2020; 141:e139–596.
2. Hong KS, Yegiaian S, Lee M, et al. Declining stroke and vascular event recurrence rates in secondary prevention trials over the past 50 years and consequences for current trial design. Circulation 2011; 123:2111–9.
3. Yang Q, Tong X, Schieb L, et al. Vital signs: recent trends in stroke death rates — United States, 2000–2015. MMWR Morb Mortal Wkly Rep 2017;66:933–9.
4. Gurol ME. Nonpharmacological management of atrial fibrillation in patients at high intracranial hemorrhage risk. Stroke 2018;49(1):247–54.
5. Kleindorfer DO, Towfighi A, Chaturvedi S, et al. 2021 Guideline for the prevention of stroke in patients with stroke and transient ischemic attack: a guideline from the American Heart Association/American Stroke Association. Stroke 2021;52(7):e364–467 [Erratum appears in Stroke 2021;52(7):e483-e484].
6. Adams HP Jr, Bendixen BH, Kappelle LJ, et al. Classification of subtype of acute ischemic stroke: definitions for use in a multicenter clinical trial. TOAST. Trial of Org 10172 in Acute Stroke Treatment. Stroke 1993;24:35–41.
7. Tsai HH, Kim JS, Jouvent E, et al. Updates on prevention of hemorrhagic and lacunar strokes. J Stroke 2018;20(2):167–79.
8. Gokcal E, Horn MJ, Gurol ME. The role of biomarkers and neuroimaging in ischemic/hemorrhagic risk assessment for cardiovascular/cerebrovascular disease prevention. Handbook Clin Neurol 2021;177:345–57.
9. Rothwell PM, Eliasziw M, Gutnikov SA, et al, Carotid Endarterectomy Trialists' Collaboration. Analysis of pooled data from the randomised controlled trials of endarterectomy for symptomatic carotid stenosis. Lancet 2003;361:107–16.
10. Brott TG, Hobson RW 2nd, Howard G, et al. CREST Investigators. Stenting versus endarterectomy for treatment of carotid-artery stenosis. N Engl J Med 2010;363:11–23.
11. Chimowitz MI, Lynn MJ, Derdeyn CP, et al. SAMMPRIS Trial Investigators. Stenting versus aggressive medical therapy for intracranial arterial stenosis. N Engl J Med 2011;365:993–1003.
12. Homma S, Thompson JL, Pullicino PM, et al, WARCEF Investigators. Warfarin and aspirin in patients with heart failure and sinus rhythm. N Engl J Med 2012;366(20):1859–69.
13. Zannad F, Anker SD, Byra WM, et al, COMMANDER HF Investigators. Rivaroxaban in patients with heart failure, sinus rhythm, and coronary disease. N Engl J Med 2018;379(14):1332–42.
14. Hart RG, Sharma M, Mundl H, et al, NAVIGATE ESUS Investigators. Rivaroxaban for stroke prevention after embolic stroke of undetermined source. N Engl J Med 2018;378:2191–201.
15. Diener HC, Sacco RL, Easton JD, et al. RE-SPECT ESUS Steering Committee and Investigators. Dabigatran for prevention of stroke after embolic stroke of undetermined source. N Engl J Med 2019;380: 1906–17.
16. Sanna T, Diener HC, Passman RS, et al, CRYSTAL AF Investigators. Cryptogenic stroke and underlying atrial fibrillation. N Engl J Med 2014;370: 2478–86.
17. Bernstein RA, Kamel H, Granger CB, et al, STROKE-AF Investigators. Effect of long-term continuous cardiac monitoring vs usual care on detection of atrial fibrillation in patients with stroke attributed to large- or small-vessel disease: the STROKE-AF Randomized Clinical Trial. JAMA 2021;325(21): 2169–77.
18. Alkhouli M, Alqahtani F, Aljohani S, et al. Burden of atrial fibrillation-associated ischemic stroke in the United States. JACC Clin Electrophysiol 2018;4: 618–25.
19. Chen LY, Chung MK, Allen LA, et al. American Heart Association Council on Clinical Cardiology; Council on Cardiovascular and Stroke Nursing; Council on Quality of Care and Outcomes Research; and Stroke Council. Atrial fibrillation burden: moving beyond atrial fibrillation as a binary entity: a scientific statement from the American

Heart Association. Circulation 2018;137(20):e623–44.

20. Wolf PA, Dawber TR, Thomas HE Jr, et al. Epidemiologic assessment of chronic atrial fibrillation and risk of stroke: the Framingham study. Neurology 1978;28(10):973–7.

21. Connolly SJ, Ezekowitz MD, Yusuf S, Eikelboom J, Oldgren J, Parekh A, Pogue J, Reilly PA, Themeles E, Varrone J, et al, RE-LY Steering Committee, Investigators. Dabigatran versus warfarin in patients with atrial fibrillation. N Engl J Med 2009; 361:1139–51.

22. Granger CB, Alexander JH, McMurray JJ, et al. ARISTOTLE Committees and Investigators. Apixaban versus warfarin in patients with atrial fibrillation. N Engl J Med 2011;365:981–92.

23. Patel MR, Mahaffey KW, Garg J, et al. ROCKET AF Investigators. Rivaroxaban versus warfarin in nonvalvular atrial fibrillation. N Engl J Med 2011;365: 883–91.

24. Seiffge DJ, De Marchis GM, Koga M, et al, RAF, RAF-DOAC, CROMIS-2, SAMURAI, NOACISP, Erlangen, and Verona registry collaborators.. Ischemic stroke despite oral anticoagulant therapy in patients with atrial fibrillation. Ann Neurol 2020; 87(5):677–87.

25. Lamassa M, Di Carlo A, Pracucci G, et al. Characteristics, outcome, and care of stroke associated with atrial fibrillation in Europe: data from a multicenter multinational hospital-based registry (the European Community Stroke Project). Stroke 2001;32:392–8.

26. Saposnik G, Gladstone D, Raptis R, et al. Atrial fibrillation in ischemic stroke: predicting response to thrombolysis and clinical outcomes. Stroke 2013;44:99–104.

27. Kimura K, Minematsu K, Yamaguchi T. Japan Multicenter Stroke Investigators; Collaboration (J-MUSIC). Atrial fibrillation as a predictive factor for severe stroke and early death in 15,831 patients with acute ischaemic stroke. J Neurol Neurosurg Psychiatr 2005;76:679–83.

28. Hayden DT, Hannon N, Callaly E, et al. Rates and determinants of 5-year outcomes after atrial fibrillation-related stroke: a population study. Stroke 2015;46(12):3488–93 [Erratum appears in Stroke 2015;46(12):e262].

29. Ali AN, Abdelhafiz A. Clinical and economic implications of AF related stroke. J Atr Fibrillation 2016; 8(5):1279.

30. Giugliano RP, Ruff CT, Braunwald E, et al. ENGAGE AF-TIMI 48 Investigators. Edoxaban versus warfarin in patients with atrial fibrillation. N Engl J Med 2013;369:2093–104.

31. Seiffge DJ, Werring DJ, Paciaroni M, et al. Timing of anticoagulation after recent ischaemic stroke in patients with atrial fibrillation. Lancet Neurol 2019; 18:117–26.

32. SoSTART Collaboration. Effects of oral anticoagulation for atrial fibrillation after spontaneous intracranial haemorrhage in the UK: a randomised, open-label, assessor-masked, pilot-phase, noninferiority trial. Lancet Neurol 2021;20(10):842–53.

33. Schreuder F, van Nieuwenhuizen KM, Hofmeijer J, APACHE-AF Trial Investigators. Apixaban versus no anticoagulation after anticoagulation-associated intracerebral haemorrhage in patients with atrial fibrillation in the Netherlands (APACHE-AF): a randomised, open-label, phase 2 trial. Lancet Neurol 2021;20(11):907–16. https://doi.org/10.1016/S1474-4422(21)00298-2.

34. Blackshear JL, Odell JA. Appendage obliteration to reduce stroke in cardiac surgical patients with atrial fibrillation. Ann Thorac Surg 1996;61(2):755–9.

35. Stoddard MF, Dawkins PR, Prince CR, et al. Left atrial appendage thrombus is not uncommon in patients with acute atrial fibrillation and a recent embolic event: a transesophageal echocardiographic study. J Am Coll Cardiol 1995;25(2):452–9.

36. Reddy VY, Doshi SK, Kar S, et al, PREVAIL and PROTECT AF Investigators. 5-year outcomes after left atrial appendage closure: from the PREVAIL and PROTECT AF trials. J Am Coll Cardiol 2017;70:2964–75.

37. Osmancik P, Herman D, Neuzil P, et al. PRAGUE-17 trial investigators. Left atrial appendage closure versus direct oral anticoagulants in high-risk patients with atrial fibrillation. J Am Coll Cardiol 2020;75(25):3122–35.

38. Kar S, Doshi SK, Sadhu A, et al, PINNACLE FLX Investigators. Primary outcome evaluation of a next-generation left atrial appendage closure device: results from the PINNACLE FLX trial. Circulation 2021;143(18):1754–62.

39. Lakkireddy D, Thaler D, Ellis CR, et al, Amulet IDE Investigators. Amplatzer Amulet left atrial appendage occluder versus Watchman device for stroke prophylaxis (Amulet IDE): a randomized controlled trial. Circulation 2021. https://doi.org/10.1161/CIRCULATIONAHA.121.057063.

40. Sposato LA, Gurol ME. Advances in neurocardiology: focus on atrial fibrillation. Stroke 2021;52(11): 3696–9.

# Left Atrial Thrombus—Are All Atria and Appendages Equal?

Alberto Cresti, MD[a], Oscar Camara, PhD[b],*

---

## KEYWORDS

- Left atrial appendage • Atrial thrombosis • Atrial fibrillation • Appendage occlusion
- Computational tools

---

## KEY POINTS

- The left atrial appendage is the main source of cardioembolic stroke, not just a useless attachment to the heart.
- Left atrial appendage morphologic variability is very high, and normal reference values are still not clearly defined.
- A multimodality imaging approach, using advanced computational tools for their exploration and analysis, is the key to better understand the left atrial appendage anatomy and function.
- The best treatment options to prevent clot formation should be personalized.

---

Video content accompanies this article at http://www.interventional.theclinics.com

## INTRODUCTION

Modern science shows how much humans are alike, with 99.9% of genome of any 2 individuals being identical. The homogeneity in human organ's structure and function is not surprising, despite the existence of variability in gender and ethnicity, among other aspects, as well as congenital malformations. Therefore, the concept of normality in healthy organs covers the normal range of variations, knowledge of which is crucial to identify abnormal patterns in anatomy and function of the studied organs.

However, there are structures in the human body that challenge the concepts of normality and standard ranges of variability, such as the left atrial appendage (LAA). The LAA is the only remnant of the primitive atrium, developing since the third gestational week[1] and has a small fingerlike size and decentralized position. The

right and LAAs seem as extensions hanging off each atrium.[2] The LAA seems apparently useless, without a clear function in adult life or a clear consequence to surgical amputation. Moreover, the LAA present an extreme range of 3-dimensional (3D) morphologic variability, as can be seen in **Fig. 1**. Can you imagine any other human structure that could be categorized as a chicken wing, a cactus, a windsock, or a cauliflower[3]? How would you define normality over all these structures? Shape variability is interesting because it is the most common site for clot formation[4] in atrial fibrillation (AF) patients and has been therefore defined as "the most lethal attachment to the heart."[5]

The mystery of the LAA has not been solved mainly due to difficulties obtaining patient-specific, robust, and quantitative metrics of anatomy and function that allow the definition of normality, which would enable thrombus risk

---

[a] Cardiology Department, Misericordia Hospital, Azienda Sanitaria Toscana SudEst, Via Senese, Grosseto 58100, Italy; [b] BCN MedTech, Department of Information and Communication Technologies, Universitat Pompeu Fabra, Tànger 122, Barcelona 08018, Spain
* Corresponding author.
E-mail address: oscar.camara@upf.edu
Twitter: @oscarcamararey (O.C.)

Intervent Cardiol Clin 11 (2022) 121–134
https://doi.org/10.1016/j.iccl.2021.11.005
2211-7458/22/© 2021 Elsevier Inc. All rights reserved.

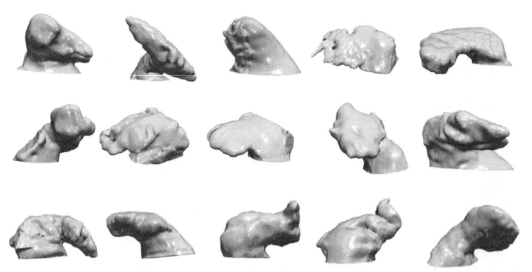

**Fig. 1.** Three-dimensional reconstructions of left atrial appendages from computer tomography scans, showing the large morphologic variability in different cases.

stratification and by extension personalize treatment. For instance, accurate LAA morphology characterization is key for selecting the optimal LAA closure device. In this paper the authors present a comprehensive review of anatomic and functional LAA differences in relation to thrombus formation and occlusion procedures, as well as the advanced imaging and computational techniques that fully characterize LAA features.

## ANATOMY
### Embryogenesis
The LAA is a remnant of the primitive atrium, with the proliferation of the mesodermal cells determining its muscular wall and pectinate muscles; the heart looping and the connection with the pulmonary veins produces variable and irregular shapes.[1] Very few developmental abnormalities of the LAA have been reported. Apart from appendage isomerism, congenital abnormalities include aplasia, hypoplasia, aneurysms, accessory appendages, and LAA membranes. Most LAA aneurysms should be operated on, as they represent risk factors for thrombosis, arrhythmias, and rupture. Less is known about hypoplasia, which may reduce thrombosis risk, and about LAA membranes, which, on the contrary, may increase it. Congenital absence of the LAA is an extremely rare cardiac anomaly, with unknown physiologic consequences.

### Left Atrial Appendage Anatomy
The LAA is attached to the anterolateral LA wall, and it is in close spatial relation with the left phrenic nerve, the left upper pulmonary vein

(LUPV), and the left circumflex artery. Only the posterior-superior border of the LAA is clearly separated from the LUPV, by a ridge (pulmonary or Coumadin ridge) that represents a remnant of the superior vena cava (Marshall ligament), whereas the other margins continue directly with the LA walls. Pits or recesses frequently surround the ostium and may contribute to thrombus formation.[6] As experience in LAAC accumulates, coverage of the pulmonary ridge is becoming relevant in the implantation of occluder devices to lower incidence of device-related thrombosis.[7]

Two appendages are present in the human heart (Fig. 2). Because of their different anatomy, the frequency of right atrial appendage (RAA) thrombi is approximately 12 times less frequent compared with LAA.[8] Although the LAA is an external structure attached to the left atrium, the right one seems as a prolongation of the right atrial cavity with a broad base. The RAA is shallow, with a single triangular lobe and a smooth surface; the "terminal crest" represents its "roof." Pectinate muscles and sagittal bands radiate from the terminal crest into the RAA, improving atrial contractility, which may play a role in preventing thrombus formation. Finally, the RAA has less plasticity, lacking significant remodeling in AF.[9]

The LAA communicates with the LA by means of an ostium (or orifice), which is narrow and well defined due to the LAA tubular shape.[10] The LAA ostium is oval shaped (69%), otherwise round, water drop–, or footlike. Wang and colleagues[3] obtained the following mean ostium dimensions: maximum diameter of 25.4 ± 5.5 mm, minimum

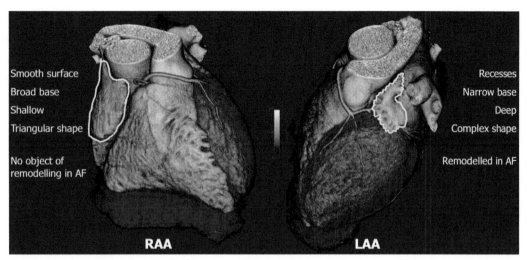

Smooth surface
Broad base
Shallow
Triangular shape

No object of
remodelling in AF

Recesses
Narrow base
Deep
Complex shape

Remodelled in AF

**RAA**                                    **LAA**

**Fig. 2.** Cardiac computed tomography showing the different characteristics of left and right appendages (LAA and RAA, respectively). AF, atrial fibrillation.

diameter of 16.8 ± 4.5 mm, and perimeter of 77.1 ± 17.9 mm. Enlargement of the LAA orifice area[11] was found an independent stroke risk factor in patients with nonvalvular AF, whereas others report the opposite.[12]

The LAA length was also estimated by Wang and colleagues[3] (45.8 ± 12.1 mm). Khurram and colleagues[12] found shorter LAA lengths being associated with stroke, whereas others[13] stated the contrary. In a similar way, Khurram and colleagues[12] did not find significant differences in LA anteroposterior diameters between controls and stroke patients, whereas others[11,13] observed larger LA dimensions in stroke cases. Table 1 summarizes the variability of different LAA features. In an autopsy study[14] a wide range of LAA volumes was found (0.7–19.2 mL). More recently, Tian and colleagues[15] estimated an LAA volume greater than 9.5 mL as a threshold to predict AF recurrence after radiofrequency ablation of the pulmonary veins.

When analyzing LA and LAA measurements, several factors influence the obtained values. First, some measurements are load dependent; volume loading increases the orifice size by an average of 1.9 mm and the LAA depth of 2.5 mm[16] (see Supplementary Material, Video 1). Second, there are discrepancies between measurements estimated from different imaging modalities. For instance, ostial size dimensions are more accurate in 3D transesophageal echocardiography (TOE) than in 2D counterparts; although a slight underestimation compared with computed tomography (CT) data is reported.[17–19]

The presence and number of secondary lobes in the LAA is variable and potentially related to thromboembolism. An LAA lobe can be defined as an outpouching of the LAA of at least 1 cm in width and depth.[20] In an autopsy study,[21] the LAA was bilobed in 54%, a single lobe was found in 20%, and 3 or more in 26%. Di Biase and colleagues[22] suggested that patients with more LAA lobes and shape complexity are significantly more likely to have emboli. Main lobe bending,[23] when the LAA presents an acute angle bend or fold from the proximal/middle portion of the LAA, has also been associated with a lower risk of embolic stroke.[24] Finally, Nedios and colleagues[25] observed a relationship between the risk of thrombus and the relative position of the LAA with the LUPV and the mitral valve.

### Left Atrial Appendage Morphology Classifications

The most commonly used LAA morphology classification was proposed by Wang and colleagues,[3] based on CT image analysis, where they qualitatively described the infamous Chicken wing (a long dominant lobe bending < 100° in its proximal part), Cactus (a central lobe < 40 mm with secondary lobes and recesses), Windsock (dominant lobe > 40 mm and secondary lobe/s bending > 100°), and Cauliflower (length < 40 mm with irregular multiple recess) categories. The same team[22] found that Chicken Wing LAA morphologies were less likely to have stroke, whereas Cactus and Cauliflower LAA were more prone to having embolic events.

However, several studies[12,25,26] have raised concerns about the robustness of this classification relating LAA morphology to thrombogenesis. First, the qualitative definitions have limited,

**Table 1**
**Variability of left atrial appendage features**

| Feature | Description | Normal Values | References |
|---|---|---|---|
| Anatomy | | | |
| Morphology | 3D conformation of the LAA | Chicken wing (48%)<br>Cactus (30%)<br>Windsock (19%)<br>Cauliflower (3%) | Di Biase 2012[22] |
| Area | Planimetric area as measured at midesophageal 2-chamber TOE view | 4.4 ± 1.1 (horizontal view)<br>3.6 ± 1.2 (vertical view) | Mügge 1994[42] |
| Volume (mL) | CT/TOE | 9.21 ± 3.18 (CT)<br>4.54 ± 1.70 (3D TOE) | Bai, 2017[18] |
| Axial orientation | The conformation and the direction along the long axis | Tip usually anterosuperior, sometimes inferior o posterior | Kanmanthareddy 2014[1] |
| Curvature | The grade of body curving | In 75% of cases, in turns 90° ± 20° after 14 ± 4 mm | Syed 2015[23] |
| Thickness | Wall thickness as measured at midesophageal 2-chamber TOE | 0.4–1.5 mm | Holmes 2009[6] |
| Lobe | The number of lobes that forms the LAA | Single lobe (20%–70%)<br>2 lobes (16%–54%)<br>3–4 lobes (remaining) | Veinot 1997,[21] Di Biase 2012[22] |
| Ostium width | Largest diameter | 16.7–21.7 mm | Nucifora 2011[17] |
| Ostium depth | The longest distance from LAA Orifice to the tip | 20–31.2 mm | Nucifora 2011[17] |
| Orifice area | MPR 3D TOE | 1.57–3.19 cm | Nucifora 2011[17] |
| Function | | | |
| Emptying velocity | The speed of emptying as assessed with pulsed Doppler | 58 ± 18 cm/s | Mügge 1994[42] |

only 28.9%, interoperator consensus.[26] Moreover, Bai and colleagues[18] found statistically significant bias in LAA morphology classification by operators presented with different imaging modalities. Some researchers have proposed a reduced list of LAA shape types improved interobserver agreement.[27] Yaghi and colleagues[24] introduced an LAA classification system based on the angle bend from the proximal/middle portion of the LAA, with greater than 90° angles being associated with higher risk of embolic stroke. In addition, statistical shape models of LAA geometries[28] automatically identified 2 distinct LAA shape clusters (Chicken Wing and non–Chicken Wing), with the LAA size, main lobe bending, and tip width being the main modes of variation.

## Gender, Ethnicity, and Interspecies Variations

Available clinical data suggest a higher thromboembolism rate in women.[29] However, Boucebci and colleagues[30] only found significant differences in LAA length and maximum width (longer in men), with a decrease of 2% in LAA ejection fraction per decade in both sexes. Kamiński and colleagues[29] observed that LAA in female populations were typically composed of 2 lobes, whereas 2- or 3-lobed appendages were most usual in the male group. In addition, they found a smaller orifice size in women, as well as a longer more tubular shape of the LAA lobes, which could explain a higher risk of thrombus formation in women.

A higher risk of cardioembolic stroke has also been reported in black people.[31] Mumin and colleagues[32] analyzed the LAA shape in Kenyan patients, finding similar prevalence of Cauliflower (the highest), Chicken Wing, and Windsock types, with Cactus being the least frequent. A basic comparison of anatomic reports[32] shows that the most common LAA shape differs by geography (Windsock predominates for Americans, Turkish, and Finish; Chicken Wing for Italians; and Cactus for Japanese). Egyptian patients preferentially have windsock LAA shapes,[33] but women seem less likely to have Chicken Wing morphology but have larger LAA volumes, smaller LAA length, and a higher prevalence of high LAA orifice position. In addition, Asians have larger LAA ostium diameters than non-Asians,[34] hence requiring larger LAAO devices. Finally, a new study[35] did not find significant differences in LA diameters/volumes or pulmonary configuration between Indigenous and non-Indigenous Australians, despite the former having a greater AF burden at younger ages. However, a tendency was observed toward non-Chicken Wing types and more eccentric, oval-shaped LAA ostia in Indigenous Australians.

All large mammals have an earlike appendage,[36] although size and shape vary considerably between species. For instance, Hill and Iaizzo[36] mainly found tubular LAA shapes in fresh ex-vivo human and canine hearts, whereas ovine and porcine LAA morphologies were rather triangular. Canine models may be useful for device testing, as their LAA have similar bending angles to human ones.[37] However, Reinthaler[38] preferred the pig model to investigate LAAO devices, as there is an underrepresentation of challenging LAA shapes in the canine model. One limitation of all these sinus rhythm models is the lack of relevance to AF; to circumvent this Olivares and colleagues[39] investigated feline models with a tendency to hypertrophic cardiomyopathy (a restrictive condition that increases the risk of AF and stroke in humans), finding similar patterns to humans when comparing cardiomyopathy cats with normals, as well as thrombus versus nonthrombus cases, that is, larger LA/LAA volumes, LAA length, and orifice areas in pathologic hearts.

## THROMBOGENESIS

### Normal Physiology

In sinus rhythm during early diastole, the LAA behaves as a conduit, whereas in late diastole (eg, atrial contraction) it assists left ventricular filling as an active contractile chamber. The LAA may act as an additional volume reservoir to the LA: it is more distensible than the left atrium, and it can be a decompression chamber when atrial pressure is increased or volume overloaded[40]; this may relate to its function as an endocrine organ, being the main site of production of atrial natriuretic peptide. Consequently, the LAA has an important role in maintaining normal fluid hemostasis; diuresis, natriuresis, and increased heart rate can be observed with elevated LAA pressures.[41]

In sinus rhythm, LAA contraction generates a positive pulse Doppler signal on echocardiography (1 cm inside the LAA ostium), representing the emptying velocity as a useful indicator of appendage contractility. Normally, LAA peak emptying velocities in sinus rhythm are greater than 50 cm/s[40], but a cutoff value of less than 40 cm/s is commonly used to define a significant reduction.[43] After LAA contraction, the filling is represented by a negative inflow signal, followed by a small systolic reflection wave.

### Pathophysiology and Thrombus Generation

LAA myopathy is defined by LAA emptying velocities less than 20 cm/s[44]. Relapse of AF is frequent with velocities less than 40 cm/s; the lower the velocity, the greater the probability of arrhythmia recurrence. In AF, pulse Doppler echocardiography signals are lost, and alternating positive and negative waves with different amplitudes are seen. By contrast, in atrial flutter a series of regular positive and negative waves of similar amplitudes are observed, with a mean velocity higher than observed in AF. However, although velocities are different between flutter and fibrillation, thrombus risk is similar,[45] suggesting there is more than slow flow to thrombus formation.

The 3 determinant factors of thrombosis were described by Virchow[46] (**Fig. 3**): (1) endothelial/endocardial damage/dysfunction and related structural changes; (2) hemodynamic changes, such as blood stasis or turbulence; and (3) increased coagulability. In AF a prothrombotic or hypercoagulable state can be caused by abnormal changes in blood flow, atrial wall, and blood components. Activation of the clotting system, oxidative stress, and inflammation may trigger atrial thrombogenesis. D-dimer, fibrinogen, platelet factor-4, and von Willebrand factor,[47] as well as C-reactive protein, interleukins, and tumor necrosis factor alpha may be elevated in AF patients, thus increasing thrombotic risk.[48] Endothelial damage/dysfunction may be imaged by cardiac magnetic resonance,[49] allowing detection of left atrium wall fibrosis that is independently associated with LAA thrombus.

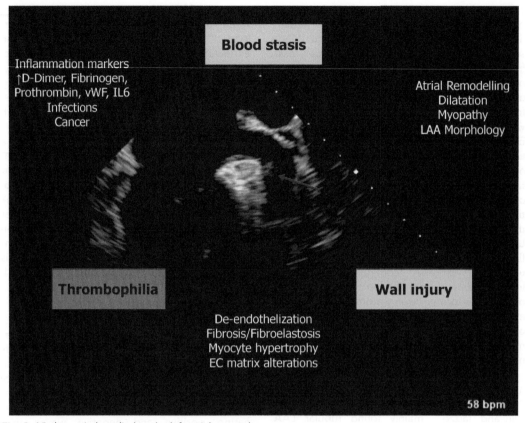

**Fig. 3.** Virchow triad applied to the left atrial appendage.

But endothelial factors, and the associated secretome, should affect the whole LA, so why in a large population of nonvalvular AF patients is the prevalence of thrombosis not localized inside the left appendage very low (0.28%)[4]? Does LAA morphology, with its deep, narrow cavity and the enlargement due to AF remodeling, the presence of acute angles, and its complex shape with multiple lobes and recesses, increase blood stasis? Although not fully established, there is evidence on the protective role of Chicken Wing LAA types (or less complex shapes) and the relevance of ostium characteristics, LAA length, main lobe bending, and LAA ejection fraction[44] in thrombus formation.

Nevertheless, LAA anatomy alone is not sufficient to fully explain thrombogenic risk; LA hemodynamics may play an important additional role. For instance, blood stasis due to mitral stenosis is a severe risk factor for atrial and appendage thrombus formation,[50] whereas mitral regurgitation, with high velocity flow inside the LA, may reverse the stasis and play a preventive role.[51]

## Improving Thrombus Risk Indices

$CHA_2DS_2$-VASc is the most widely used stroke risk stratification score in AF patients but has limited value to identify at-risk patients for several reasons. First, although it includes some clinical factors it ignores, others, for example, paroxysmal versus permanent AF, have the same significance. Other missing parameters that generally confer thrombotic risk include chronic kidney disease, obesity, sedentary lifestyle, obstructive sleep apnea syndrome, and the type and severity of underlying heart disease. In addition, LA/LAA morphologic and functional characteristics or biomarkers such as proB-type natriuretic peptide or troponin are absent.

LAA emptying velocities, although an expression of appendage myopathy and thrombosis risk, poorly correlate with LA anatomic and functional variables and should not be used as surrogates of global LA function.[52] To better evaluate LAA function and thrombogenic risk, additional imaging parameters have been evaluated, such as the LAA ejection fraction.[18] Reduced LAA contractility, measured by speckle-tracking echocardiography, E/e' and e' velocity, as well as LA strain, are new methodologies that have been found to independently correlate with LAA thrombus in nonvalvular AF. Currently, these are not routinely used to assess LA performance, and inferring LAA thrombotic risk, due to difficulties in defining appendage boundaries and ostium dimensions, in addition to absence of technical standards and normal reference values.

Improving patient thrombotic stratification could come from advanced morphologic and functional indices of the LA and LAA, as well as clinically relevant information. For instance, Mill and colleagues[53] jointly analyzed CT-based morphologic and in-silico hemodynamics metrics to study the influence of the PV configuration on LA blood flow, obtaining differences in LAA washout for non–Chicken Wing morphologies with and without stroke history. Unfortunately, most of these indices can only be extracted in a robust way with sophisticated imaging systems and computational tools that are not available for routine clinical use yet.

## INSTRUMENTATION/IMPLANTATION

For patients with contraindications to oral anticoagulants, LAAO implantation is becoming accepted. Several devices are available in the market (eg, Amulet-Amplatzer, Watchman (FLX), LAmbre, WaveCrest, Ultraseal), all providing different sizes, with new products continuously being developed (eg, CLASS, OMEGA, Occlutech Plus, etc.). Clinicians need to decide which type of device to implant, which size (also considering acceptable ranges of overcompression), and the optimal position (definition of landing zone) to avoid leaks, embolization, and device-related thrombus (DRT) after the intervention.

The optimal LAAO device implantation reflects LAA anatomic variability and is necessarily different for each patient. Dimensions of the ostium (and how oval it is), LAA depth and width, the landing zone, the circumflex position, the distance of the LAA to the pulmonary ridge and mitral valve, and the presence and angle of LAA bending, trabeculations or secondary lobes next to the ostium, need to be considered during device selection. These indices can generally be extracted from multimodal medical images, but caution is needed due to discrepancies in measurements from distinct imaging techniques; López-Minguez and colleagues[54] found consistent device sizing for LAA closure in only 21.6% of the cases when using CT, TOE, and angiography images.

Fortunately, the success rates of LAAO implantation is very high (eg, 98.6% in a recent study[7]), but suboptimal LAAO selection may contribute to a nonnegligible number of adverse events such as DRT (Fauchier and colleagues[55] reported from 5.5% to 11% in real-world clinical data). For instance, the relevance of covering the pulmonary ridge to avoid DRT was recently reported.[7,56] **Fig. 4** shows the use of in-silico simulations to identify differences in blood flow patterns covering or not covering the pulmonary ridge prior knowledge of which may influence device choice or shared-decision making discussions with patients or their families.

Additional time and effort spent determining thrombotic risk pre-/postdevice will also pick out the rare LAA morphologies that are harder to close, especially those with irregular ostium shapes, very large dimensions, small necks, high bending close to the ostium, or LAA position far from the pulmonary ridge and close to the mitral valve. For some complex cases, less commonly used LAAO devices (eg, LAmbre or CLAAS) might be appropriate. The sandwich technique can be used in the Chicken Wing LAA with severe bending short necks[57] that is hostile to plug-type devices.

Since complications associated to LAAC are non-negligible, it is important to identify the patients who will benefit more from the LAA closure. It is still unclear if there are long-term effects from "removing" a cavity in the LA. Some studies have suggested heart failure deterioration may be caused by LAA exclusion,[58] due to the reduction of atrial and brain natriuretic peptide secretion. In addition, several animal experiments[59] show LAA removal led to reduction in left atrial compliance (and thus, reservoir function), cardiac output, stroke volume, and even water retention, all factors that could promote heart decompensation, particularly those with restrictive physiology.

Conceptually LAAC and OAC are not managing embolic stroke risk in the same way. The key difference is that LAA closure targets the flow factor of Virchow's triad, whereas OAC addresses thrombogenicity. Optimal treatment of a given patient should consider which factors are more relevant and find the most appropriate combination of drug and device therapies to maximize benefit and minimize risk. For instance, a complex LAA morphology, where the pulmonary ridge will not be covered, in a highly thrombogenic patient, could require continuous OAC to avoid DRT, making LAAO more a problem than a solution. Conversely, simpler slow flow LAA morphologies in patients

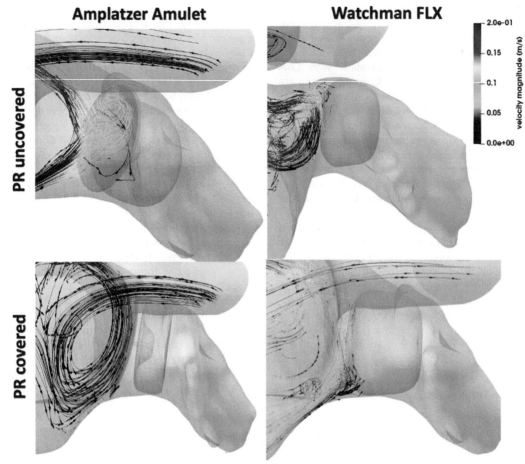

**Fig. 4.** In-silico fluid simulations with 2 different left atrial occluder devices in 2 distinct positions, with the pulmonary ridge (PR) covered and uncovered. The coverage of the PR leads to higher blood flow velocities and more laminar flows.

with high bleeding risk would be more suitable for LAAO as a first-line treatment.

## FUTURE DEVELOPMENTS
### Multimodal Imaging
In most clinical centers, echocardiography, mainly transthoracic preprocedural and transesophageal (TOE) during the procedure, is used for planning and guiding the LAAO implantation, together with radiographic fluoroscopy. Both imaging techniques allow real-time visualization of the LA anatomy and dynamics during the intervention, showing the status of the patient at the time of the procedure and the relation with the implanted device. However, the poor image resolution and the 2D nature of these 2 modalities hamper a full characterization of the LAA anatomy. Furthermore, Doppler data provide oversimplified indices of the complex 4D nature of blood flow. New echocardiographic systems that eliminate the need for general anesthesia in LAAO procedures, such as

intracardiac echocardiography[60] or transnasal TOE,[61] retain many of the imaging limitations and require interventional imaging skills and more cost-efficiency studies to prove their added value.

CT is emerging as a valid alternative for preprocedural planning and follow-up,[62] providing excellent 3D image resolution that permits a more robust morphologic analysis, improving device selection accuracy and reducing procedural time. However, CT has a poor positive predictive value (41%) for detection of LAA thrombus[63] in standard acquisitions. Contrast delayed imaging or use of dual-energy CT may help to differentiate between poor LAA filling or thrombosis.[64] Postprocedure CT still overestimates the occurrence of peri-device leaks compared with TOE.[65] Cardiac MRI has also been used to identify the presence of LAA thrombus, with a high concordance with TOE,[66] with the additional potential of measuring LAA flow. Indeed, advanced imaging techniques to better characterize blood flow

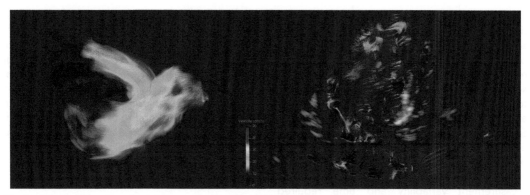

Fig. 5. Advanced imaging modalities to visualize blood flow patterns and velocities in the left atria. (*Left*) 4D flow magnetic resonance imaging. (*Right*) Blood speckle imaging.

patterns such as 4D flow MRI and blood speckle imaging, are starting to be adapted to the left atria[67,68] (**Fig. 5** and Supplementary Material, Video 2 and Video 3).

### Advanced Computational Tools
Medical images of the LAA are usually rendered as multiplanar reconstructions visualized on a 2D screen, making it difficult to capture the 3D nature of the LAA. Moreover, measurements of LAA morphology are obtained manually, which is prone to high intra- and interobserver variability, especially in noisy images such as echocardiography and radiographs. However, LAA-tailored software such as 3mensio Structural Heart software (Pie Medical Imaging, Bilthoven, the Netherlands) and Materialise Mimics (NV, Leuven, Belgium) already include advanced visualization tools such as 3D rendering, landing zone assessment, automatic LAA measurements,

simulation of radiographs, virtual device implantation and manipulation, as well as planning of transeptal puncture. The VIDAA research platform[69] is a web-based alternative that also allows a full characterization of the LAA morphology and the virtual implantation and manipulation of devices recommended based on the LAA morphologic analysis (**Fig. 6** and Supplementary Material, Video 4).

Advanced rendering tools also improve our understanding of LAA anatomy. For instance, tissue transparency transillumination facilitates delineation of cardiac structures, including the LAA, when analyzing 3D echocardiographic images.[70] Cinematic rendering has also been proposed for generating photorealistic illustrations of the cardiac anatomy from CT images.[71] Moreover, multimodal fusion of echocardiographic and radiographic images during the intervention reduces procedural times and contrast use.[72]

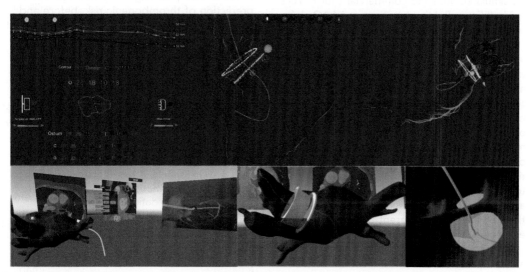

Fig. 6. Advanced visualization platforms for the morphologic analysis of the left atria and virtual implantation of occluder devices. (*Top*) Web-based VIDAA platform. (*Bottom*) Virtual reality VRIDAA platform.

The aforementioned imaging and visualization techniques are still limited to 2D flat screens, hampering the scaling and depth perception required to fully understand the 3D nature of the LAA. Augmented or virtual reality solutions, as well as 3D printing, may be used for further exploration of left atrial anatomy and better planning of LAAO interventions. Several studies have evaluated the added value of 3D printed models for training and planning of LAAO interventions.[73] Narang and colleagues[74] recently demonstrated a reduction in measurement variability and time required when exploring with a VR system cardiac structures such as the LAA. Also, the VRIDAA platform[75] (see **Fig. 6** and Supplementary Material, Video 5) allows the visualization/analysis of LAA anatomies with the most appropriate occlusion devices to be implanted with VR headsets. Similarly, augmented/mixed reality systems are emerging with the same objective.[76]

In-silico simulations can provide a complete analysis of LA hemodynamics based on a Digital Twin built from patient-specific data. Computational fluid dynamics can be used to better understand the most relevant factors that guide blood flow patterns in the LA. The same technique can also analyze thrombus generation in the LA,[77–79] identifying regions with low velocities, recirculations or vortices, abnormal wall-shear stresses, and the relevance of PV configuration.[80] Finally, some studies[56,69] also included LAAO devices with different settings in in-silico fluid simulations, demonstrating the benefit of appropriate sizing and positioning to avoid regions prone to DRT, as shown in **Fig. 4**. Device deployment can also be simulated with the commercial tool HEART-guide (FEops, Belgium) to predict LAAO deformation and apposition.[81]

Artificial intelligence (AI) and machine learning (ML) have a major impact in radiology tasks, contributing to automating and accelerating tasks that are key for LAA-based decisions.[82] Deep learning algorithms have already been applied for the automatic segmentation of LA and LAA from CT images.[83] In addition, more recent advanced ML techniques are being developed to provide surrogates of fluid simulations[84] at almost real time. These AI-based tools, together with clinical-friendly interfaces will soon allow the interactive and fast estimation of thrombus risk with different LAAO settings for enhanced preprocedural planning.

The clinical translation of the advanced imaging and computational tools listed earlier is still challenging, requiring further development to reduce cost and simplify usage, in a clinical environment, but they certainly have a role in structural heart disease applications.[73] Recently, a comparative study performed at Universitat Pompeu Fabra, where several cardiologists tested different tools for LAAO preprocedural planning, suggested that 3D visualization including interactive manipulation of LAAO devices in conjunction with 3D printing can already be integrated in most hospitals, adding value for planning, whereas in-silico simulations could be interesting for follow-up analysis.

## SUMMARY

Arguably, we could affirm that all atria and appendages are rather different than equal, between patients due to the high morphologic variation, and even in the same person from the unclear role in health to a lethal player in disease. Why evolution left such an auricle in the left atrium in all mammals is still a mystery that needs to be elucidated, especially in relation to pathophysiological mechanisms leading to thrombus.

Despite the attempts of researchers to classify LAA morphology into nonoverlapping categories, a continuum of shapes, number of lobes, recesses, and angulations is the norm. We could say that "Nature does not know about classification," but there is enough literature showing more complex LAA anatomies are associated with higher thrombotic risk. Consequently, there is a need for quantitative metrics (eg, beyond chicken wings and vegetables) for the robust characterization of LAA anatomic and functional variations with advanced imaging and computational techniques that make more personalized planning of LAAO interventions, prediction of thrombogenic risk, before and after the procedure, and tailored follow-up treatment. The (LAA) quest continues.

## CLINICS CARE POINTS

- The LAA is the main source of cardioembolic stroke, not just a useless attachment to the heart.
- LAA anatomic and morphologic variability is very high, and normal reference values are still not clearly defined.
- A multimodality imaging approach, using advanced computational tools for their exploration and analysis, is the key to better understand the LAA anatomy and function.
- The risk of clot formation is not only a consequence of anatomic features but

depends also on global heart function and thrombophilic state.

- The study of flow dynamics and the development of new computational technologies will allow a better understanding of LAA characteristics to individualize the prevention of clot formation and embolism.

## DISCLOSURE

This work was supported by the Spanish Ministry of Economy and Competitiveness under the Retos Investigacion project (RTI2018-101193-B-I00) and by the H2020 EU SimCardioTest project (Digital transformation in Health and Care SC1-DTH-06-2020; grant agreement No. 101016496)..

## SUPPLEMENTARY DATA

Supplementary data related to this article can be found online at https://doi.org/10.1016/j.iccl.2021.11.005

## REFERENCES

1. Kanmanthareddy A, Reddy YM, Vallakati A, et al. Embryology and anatomy of the left atrial appendage: why does thrombus form? Interv Cardiol Clin 2014;3(2):191–202.
2. Iaizzo PA. Handbook of cardiac anatomy, physiology, and devices. 3rd edition. Switzerland: Springer International Publishing; 2015.
3. Wang Y, Di Biase L, Horton RP, et al. Left atrial appendage studied by computed tomography to help planning for appendage closure device placement. J Cardiovasc Electrophysiol 2010;21(9):973–82.
4. Cresti A, García-Fernández MA, Sievert H, et al. Prevalence of extra-appendage thrombosis in non-valvular atrial fibrillation and atrial flutter in patients undergoing cardioversion: a large transoesophageal echo study. EuroIntervention 2019;15(3):e225–30.
5. Johnson WD, Ganjoo AK, Stone CD, et al. The left atrial appendage: Our most lethal human attachment! Surgical implications. Eur J Cardio-thoracic Surg 2000;17(6):718–22.
6. Holmes DR, Schwartz RS. Left atrial appendage occlusion eliminates the need for warfarin. Circulation 2009;120(19):1919–26.
7. Freixa X, Cepas-Guillen P, Flores-Umanzor E, et al. Pulmonary ridge coverage and device-related thrombosis after left atrial appendage occlusion. EuroIntervention 2021;16(15):E1288–94.
8. Cresti A, García-Fernández MA, Miracapillo G, et al. Frequency and significance of right atrial appendage thrombi in patients with persistent atrial fibrillation or atrial flutter. J Am Soc Echocardiogr 2014;27(11):1200–7.
9. Subramaniam B, Riley MF, Panzica PJ, et al. Transesophageal echocardiographic assessment of right atrial appendage anatomy and function: comparison with the left atrial appendage and implications for local thrombus formation. J Am Soc Echocardiogr 2006;19(4):429–33.
10. Ho SY, Anderson RH, Sánchez-Quintana D. Atrial structure and fibres: morphologic bases of atrial conduction. Cardiovasc Res 2002;54(2):325–36.
11. Lee JM, Shim J, Uhm JS, et al. Impact of increased orifice size and decreased flow velocity of left atrial appendage on stroke in nonvalvular atrial fibrillation. Am J Cardiol 2014;113(6):963–9.
12. Khurram IM, Dewire J, Mager M, et al. Relationship between left atrial appendage morphology and stroke in patients with atrial fibrillation. Hear Rhythm 2013;10(12):1843–9.
13. Lee JM, Kim JB, Uhm JS, et al. Additional value of left atrial appendage geometry and hemodynamics when considering anticoagulation strategy in patients with atrial fibrillation with low CHA2DS2-VASc scores. Hear Rhythm 2017;14(9):1297–301.
14. Ernst G, Stöllberger C, Abzieher F, et al. Morphology of the left atrial appendage. Anat Rec 1995;242(4):553–61.
15. Tian X, Zhang XJ, Yuan YF, et al. Morphological and functional parameters of left atrial appendage play a greater role in atrial fibrillation relapse after radiofrequency ablation. Sci Rep 2020;10(1):1–10.
16. Spencer RJ, Dejong P, Fahmy P, et al. Changes in left atrial appendage dimensions following volume loading during percutaneous left atrial appendage closure. JACC Cardiovasc Interv 2015;8(15):1935–41.
17. Nucifora G, Faletra FF, Regoli F, et al. Evaluation of the left atrial appendage with real-time 3-dimensional transesophageal echocardiography implications for catheter-based left atrial appendage closure. Circ Cardiovasc Imaging 2011;4(5):514–23.
18. Bai W, Chen Z, Tang H, et al. Assessment of the left atrial appendage structure and morphology: comparison of real-time three-dimensional transesophageal echocardiography and computed tomography. Int J Cardiovasc Imaging 2017;33(5):623–33.
19. Meltzer SN, Phatak PM, Fazlalizadeh H, et al. Three-dimensional echocardiographic left atrial appendage volumetric analysis. J Am Soc Echocardiogr 2021;20010:1–9.
20. Budge LP, Shaffer KM, Moorman JR, et al. Analysis of in vivo left atrial appendage morphology in patients with atrial fibrillation: a direct comparison of

transesophageal echocardiography, planar cardiac CT, and segmented three-dimensional cardiac CT. J Interv Card Electrophysiol 2008;23(2):87–93.

21. Veinot JP, Harrity PJ, Gentile F, et al. Anatomy of the normal left atrial appendage: a quantitative study of age-related changes in 500 autopsy hearts: implications for echocardiographic examination. Circulation 1997;96(9):3112–5.

22. Di Biase L, Santangeli P, Anselmino M, et al. Does the left atrial appendage morphology correlate with the risk of stroke in patients with atrial fibrillation? Results from a multicenter study. J Am Coll Cardiol 2012;60(6):531–8.

23. Syed FF, Noheria A, De Simone CV, et al. Left atrial appendage ligation and exclusion technology in the incubator. J Atr Fibrillation 2015;8(2):61–70.

24. Yaghi S, Chang AD, Akiki R, et al. The left atrial appendage morphology is associated with embolic stroke subtypes using a simple classification system: a proof of concept study. J Cardiovasc Comput Tomogr 2020;14(1):27–33.

25. Nedios S, Kornej J, Koutalas E, et al. Left atrial appendage morphology and thromboembolic risk after catheter ablation for atrial fibrillation. Hear Rhythm 2014;11(12):2239–46.

26. Wu L, Liang E, Fan S, et al. Relation of left atrial appendage morphology determined by computed tomography to prior stroke or to increased risk of stroke in patients with atrial fibrillation. Am J Cardiol 2019;123(8):1283–6.

27. Słodowska K, Szczepanek E, Dudkiewicz D, et al. Morphology of the left atrial appendage: introduction of a new simplified shape-based classification system. Hear Lung Circ 2021;(February):31–4.

28. Slipsager JM, Juhl KA, Sigvardsen PE, et al. Statistical shape clustering of left atrial appendages. In: Pop, et al, editors. Lecture notes in computer science (including subseries lecture notes in artificial intelligence and lecture notes in bioinformatics) Vol 11395 LNCS. Switzerland: Springer Verlag; 2019. p. 32–9.

29. Kamiński R, Kosiński A, Brala M, et al. Variability of the left atrial appendage in human hearts. PLoS One 2015;10(11):1–9.

30. Boucebci S, Pambrun T, Velasco S, et al. Assessment of normal left atrial appendage anatomy and function over gender and ages by dynamic cardiac CT. Eur Radiol 2016;26(5):1512–20.

31. White H, Boden-Albala B, Wang C, et al. Ischemic stroke subtype incidence among whites, blacks, and Hispanics: The northern Manhattan study. In: CirculationVol 111. Lippincott Williams & Wilkins; 2005. p. 1327–31.

32. Mumin A, Olabu B, Kaisha W, et al. Morphology of the left atrial appendage: prevalence and gender difference in a Kenyan population. J Morphol Sci 2018;35(1):48–53.

33. Elzeneini M, Elshazly A, Nayel AEM. The left atrial appendage morphology and gender differences by multi-detector computed tomography in an Egyptian population. Egypt Hear J 2020;72(1):2–7.

34. Ono S, Kubo S, Maruo T, et al. Left atrial appendage size in patients with atrial fibrillation in Japan and the United States. Heart Vessels 2021;36(2):277–84.

35. Clarke NAR, Kangaharan N, Costello B, et al. Left atrial, pulmonary vein, and left atrial appendage anatomy in Indigenous individuals: Implications for atrial fibrillation. IJC Hear Vasc 2021;34: 100775.

36. Hill AJ, Iaizzo PA. Comparative cardiac anatomy. In: Iaizzo, et al, editors. Handbook of cardiac anatomy, physiology, and devices. 3rd edition. Switzerland: Springer International Publishing; 2015. p. 89–114.

37. Bass JL. Transcatheter occlusion of the left atrial appendage-experimental testing of a new amplatzer device. Catheter Cardiovasc Interv 2010;76(2):181–5.

38. Reinthaler M, Grosshauser J, Schmidt T, et al. Preclinical assessment of a modified Occlutech left atrial appendage closure device in a porcine model. Sci Rep 2021;11(1):1–12.

39. Olivares AL, Pons MI, Mill J, et al. Shape Analysis and Computational Fluid Simulations to Assess Feline Left Atrial Function and Thrombogenesis. In: Ennis DB, Perotti LE, Wang VY, editors. Functional Imaging and Modeling of the Heart. FIMH 2021. Lecture Notes in Computer Science, 12738. Cham, Switzerland: Springer; 2021.

40. Tabata T, Oki T, Yamada H, et al. Role of left atrial appendage in left atrial reservoir function as evaluated by left atrial appendage clamping during cardiac surgery. Am J Cardiol 1998;81(3):327–32.

41. Kappagoda CT, Linden RJ, Snow HM. The effect of distending the atrial appendages on urine flow in the dog. J Physiol 1972;227(1):233–42.

42. Mügge A, Kühn H, Nikutta P, et al. Assessment of left atrial appendage function by biplane transesophageal echocardiography in patients with nonrheumatic atrial fibrillation: Identification of a subgroup of patients at increased embolic risk. J Am Coll Cardiol 1994;23(3):599–607.

43. Fatkin D, Kelly RP, Feneley MP. Relations between left atrial appendage blood flow velocity, spontaneous echocardiographic contrast and thromboembolic risk in vivo. J Am Coll Cardiol 1994;23(4):961–9.

44. García-Fernández MA, Torrecilla EG, Román DS, et al. Left atrial appendage doppler flow patterns: implications on thrombus formation. Am Heart J 1992;124(4):955–61.

45. Cresti A, García-Fernández MA, De Sensi F, et al. Prevalence of auricular thrombosis before atrial flutter cardioversion: a 17-year transoesophageal echocardiographic study. Europace 2016;18(3): 450–6.

46. Watson T, Shantsila E, Lip GY. Mechanisms of thrombogenesis in atrial fibrillation: Virchow's triad revisited. Lancet 2009;373(9658):155–66.

47. Ohara K, Inoue H, Nozawa T, et al. Accumulation of risk factors enhances the prothrombotic state in atrial fibrillation. Int J Cardiol 2008;126(3):316–21.

48. Guo Y, Lip GYH, Apostolakis S. Inflammation in atrial fibrillation. J Am Coll Cardiol 2012;60(22): 2263–70.

49. Akoum N, Fernandez G, Wilson B, et al. Association of atrial fibrosis quantified using LGE-MRI with atrial appendage thrombus and spontaneous contrast on transesophageal echocardiography in patients with atrial fibrillation. J Cardiovasc Electrophysiol 2013;24(10):1104–9.

50. Salem DN, Stein PD, Al-Ahmad A, et al. Antithrombotic therapy in valvular heart disease - Native and prosthetic: the Seventh ACCP Conference on Antithrombotic and Thrombolytic Therapy. In: ChestVol 126. American College of Chest Physicians; 2004. p. 457S–82S.

51. Cresti A, Galli CA, Alimento ML, et al. Does mitral regurgitation reduce the risks of thrombosis in atrial fibrillation and flutter? J Cardiovasc Med (Hagerstown) 2019;20(10):660–6.

52. Agmon Y, Khandheria BK, Meissner I, et al. Are left atrial appendage flow velocities adequate surrogates of global left atrial function? A population-based transthoracic and transesophageal echocardiographic study. J Am Soc Echocardiogr 2002;15(5):433–40.

53. Mill J, Harrison J, Legghe B, et al. Large in-silico analysis of the influence of pulmonary veins ' configuration on left atrial haemodynamics and thrombus formation. In: Functional imaging and modeling of the heart. ; 2021:1-8.

54. López-Mínguez JR, González-Fernández R, Fernández-Vegas C, et al. Anatomical classification of left atrial appendages in specimens applicable to CT imaging techniques for implantation of amplatzer cardiac plug. J Cardiovasc Electrophysiol 2014; 25(9):976–84.

55. Fauchier L, Cinaud A, Brigadeau F, et al. Device-related thrombosis after percutaneous left atrial appendage occlusion for atrial fibrillation. J Am Coll Cardiol 2018;71(14):1528–36.

56. Mill J, Olivares AL, Arzamendi D, et al. Impact of flow dynamics on device-related thrombosis after left atrial appendage occlusion. Can J Cardiol 2020;36(6):968.e13–4.

57. Freixa X, Tzikas A, Aminian A, et al. Left atrial appendage occlusion in chicken-wing anatomies: imaging assessment, procedural, and clinical outcomes of the "sandwich technique.". Catheter Cardiovasc Interv 2021;97(7):E1025–32.

58. Schneider B, Nazarenus D, Stöllberger C. A 79-year-old woman with atrial fibrillation and new onset of heart failure. ESC Hear Fail 2019;6(3):570–4.

59. Stöllberger C, Schneider B, Finsterer J. Elimination of the left atrial appendage to prevent stroke or embolism? Anatomic, physiologic, and pathophysiologic considerations. Chest 2003;124(6): 2356–62.

60. Berti S, Paradossi U, Meucci F, et al. Periprocedural intracardiac echocardiography for left atrial appendage closure: a dual-center experience. JACC Cardiovasc Interv 2014;7(9):1036–44.

61. Wang B, Zhang L, Sun W, et al. Transnasal transesophageal echocardiography guidance for percutaneous left atrial appendage closure. Ann Thorac Surg 2019;108(3):e161–4.

62. Korsholm K, Berti S, Iriart X, et al. Expert recommendations on cardiac computed tomography for planning transcatheter left atrial appendage occlusion. JACC Cardiovasc Interv 2020;13(3):277–92.

63. Romero J, Husain SA, Kelesidis I, et al. Detection of left atrial appendage thrombus by cardiac computed tomography in patients with atrial fibrillation: a meta-analysis. Circ Cardiovasc Imaging 2013;6(2):185–94.

64. Hur J, Kim YJ, Lee HJ, et al. Cardioembolic stroke: dual-energy cardiac CT for differentiation of left atrial appendage thrombus and circulatory stasis. Radiology 2012;263(3):688–95.

65. Korsholm K, Jensen JM, Nørgaard BL, et al. Peridevice leak following amplatzer left atrial appendage occlusion: cardiac computed tomography classification and clinical outcomes. JACC Cardiovasc Interv 2021;14(1):83–93.

66. Ohyama H, Hosomi N, Takahashi T, et al. Comparison of magnetic resonance imaging and transesophageal echocardiography in detection of thrombus in the left atrial appendage. Stroke 2003;34(10):2436–9.

67. Markl M, Lee DC, Ng J, et al. Left atrial 4-dimensional flow magnetic resonance imaging stasis and velocity mapping in patients with atrial fibrillation. Invest Radiol 2016;51(3):147–54.

68. Morales X, Mill J, Delso G, et al. 4D flow magnetic resonance imaging for left atrial haemodynamic characterization and model calibration. In: Puyol Anton, et al, editors. Lecture notes in computer science (including subseries lecture notes in artificial intelligence and lecture notes in bioinformatics) Vol 12592 LNCS. Switzerland: Springer International Publishing; 2021. p. 156–65.

69. Aguado AM, Olivares AL, Yagüe C, et al. In silico optimization of left atrial appendage occluder implantation using interactive and modeling tools. Front Physiol 2019;10(MAR):237.

70. Karagodin I, Addetia K, Singh A, et al. Improved delineation of cardiac pathology using a novel three-dimensional echocardiographic tissue transparency tool. J Am Soc Echocardiogr 2020;33(11): 1316–23.

71. Rowe SP, Johnson PT, Fishman EK. Cinematic rendering of cardiac CT volumetric data: Principles and initial observations. J Cardiovasc Comput Tomogr 2018;12(1):56–9.

72. Ebelt H, Domagala T, Offhaus A, et al. Fusion Imaging of X-ray and transesophageal echocardiography improves the procedure of left atrial appendage closure. Cardiovasc Drugs Ther 2020; 34(6):781–7.

73. Wang DD, Qian Z, Vukicevic M, et al. 3D printing, computational modeling, and artificial intelligence for Structural Heart Disease. JACC Cardiovasc Imaging 2021;14(1):41–60.

74. Narang A, Hitschrich N, Mor-Avi V, et al. Virtual reality analysis of three-dimensional echocardiographic and cardiac computed tomographic data sets. J Am Soc Echocardiogr 2020;33(11):1306–15.

75. Medina E, Aguado AM, Mill J, et al. VRIDAA: virtual reality platform for training and planning implantations of occluder devices in left atrial appendages. Eurographics Work Vis Comput Biol Med 2020;31–5.

76. Pappalardo O, Pasquali M, Maltagliati A, et al. A platform for real-3d visualization and planning of left atrial appendage occlusion through mixed reality. Eur Hear J - Cardiovasc Imaging 2021;22(Supplement_1).

77. Bosi GM, Cook A, Rai R, et al. Computational fluid dynamic analysis of the left atrial appendage to predict thrombosis risk. Front Cardiovasc Med 2018;5.

78. Masci A, Barone L, Dedè L, et al. The impact of left atrium appendage morphology on stroke risk assessment in atrial fibrillation: A Computational Fluid Dynamics Study. Front Physiol 2019;9:1938.

79. García-Villalba M, Rossini L, Gonzalo A, et al. Demonstration of patient-specific simulations to assess left atrial appendage thrombogenesis risk. Front Physiol 2021;12.

80. García-Isla G, Olivares AL, Silva E, et al. Sensitivity analysis of geometrical parameters to study haemodynamics and thrombus formation in the left atrial appendage. Int J Numer Method Biomed Eng 2018;34(8):e3100.

81. Bavo AM, Wilkins BT, Garot P, et al. Validation of a computational model aiming to optimize preprocedural planning in percutaneous left atrial appendage closure. J Cardiovasc Comput Tomogr 2020;14(2):149–54.

82. Ribeiro JM, Astudillo P, de Backer O, et al. Artificial intelligence and transcatheter interventions for Structural Heart Disease: a glance at the (near) future. Trends Cardiovasc Med 2021. https://doi.org/10.1016/j.tcm.2021.02.002.

83. Jin C, Feng J, Wang L, et al. Left atrial appendage segmentation using fully convolutional neural networks and modified three-dimensional conditional random fields. IEEE J Biomed Heal Inform 2018; 22(6):1906–16.

84. Morales Ferez X, Mill J, Juhl KA. Deep Learning Framework for Real-Time Estimation of in-silico Thrombotic Risk Indices in the Left Atrial Appendage. Frontiers in Physiology 2021; 12(694945).

# Left Atrial Appendage Occlusion—A Choice or a Last Resort? How to Approach the Patient

Wern Yew Ding, MRCP[a], Gregory Y.H. Lip, MD[a,b], Dhiraj Gupta, MD[a,*]

## KEYWORDS

- Left atrial appendage • Occlusion • Closure • Patient choice • Anticoagulation
- Atrial fibrillation

## KEY POINTS

- There are practical challenges to the use of oral anticoagulation, including patient noncompliance, major bleeding, side effects, drug-drug interactions, and very high short-term discontinuation rates.
- Left atrial appendage occlusion is emerging as a possible alternative to oral anticoagulation in high-risk patients with atrial fibrillation.
- Left atrial appendage occlusion may be considered in patients with an absolute contraindication to and no other requirement for long-term anticoagulation; relative contraindications to anticoagulation; resistant stroke; poor quality of anticoagulation control; drug-drug interactions; or severe side effects to oral anticoagulation.

## INTRODUCTION

Atrial fibrillation (AF) is a multisystemic condition that is characterized by a prothrombotic state due to disruption of physiologic hemostatic mechanisms, best explained using Virchow triad of deranged blood constituents, vessel wall abnormalities, and blood stasis.[1] Hence, patients with AF are exposed to an increased risk of thromboembolism that may manifest as stroke. Based on current international guidelines, the use of oral anticoagulation (OAC) to reduce the risk of thromboembolic complications is recommended in non–low-risk patients with AF.[2–5]

Despite the established benefits of OAC, there remains practical challenges to the use of these medications, including patient noncompliance, major bleeding, side effects, and drug-drug interactions. Furthermore, approximately 1 in 10 patients are deemed to have a contraindication to anticoagulation, with 2% having absolute contraindications.[6,7] The issues with anticoagulation are reflected by a high discontinuation rate of up to 47% within 2 years of initiating treatment,[8] although less with non–vitamin K antagonist oral anticoagulants (NOAC).[9,10] As a result, close to 40% of real-world patients with AF who have a significant risk of stroke remain untreated,[11] rendering the quest for better treatment options an important one; this is despite efforts to improve prescription rates for OAC in patients with AF.[12]

Observational studies have shown that the left atrial appendage (LAA) is the predominant

[a] Liverpool Centre for Cardiovascular Science, University of Liverpool and Liverpool Heart & Chest Hospital, Liverpool, UK; [b] Aalborg Thrombosis Research Unit, Department of Clinical Medicine, Aalborg University, Aalborg, Denmark
* Corresponding author. Department of Cardiology, Liverpool Heart and Chest Hospital, Thomas Drive, Liverpool L14 3PE, United Kingdom
E-mail address: Dhiraj.Gupta@lhch.nhs.uk

Intervent Cardiol Clin 11 (2022) 135–142
https://doi.org/10.1016/j.iccl.2021.11.006
2211-7458/22/© 2022 Elsevier Inc. All rights reserved.

site for up to 91% of thrombus formation in patients with AF.[13–15] Thus, it has been postulated that exclusion of this anatomic structure from the circulatory system may significantly negate the risk of thromboembolic complications. In this regard, LAA occlusion has been proposed as a potential alternative to OAC in AF.[16–19]

Previously, Piccini and colleagues suggested that LAA occlusion should be reserved only for patients with a high-risk of stroke and contraindications to long-term OAC.[20] However, this viewpoint remains a topic of debate. Contemporary data from the United States showed that the clinical uptake of LAA occlusion increased significantly by 10-fold from 2015 to 2017.[21] As such, patient selection is an important issue to address. Herein, we discuss arguments for LAA occlusion as either a last resort versus patient choice and discuss practical steps in the approach of patients who may be suitable for LAA occlusion.

## LEFT ATRIAL APPENDAGE OCCLUSION AS A LAST RESORT?

In many centers, LAA occlusion remains a last resort option for patients with AF who need but are unable to tolerate long-term OAC due to absolute contraindications[2,22]; this is predicated somewhat by divergent results from the regulatory trials, relatively scarce data on the long-term efficacy and safety of LAA occlusion, concerns over the pathophysiological basis by which LAA occlusion reduces the risk of thromboembolic complications, and the widespread availability of NOAC agents.

Although the PROTECT AF trial reported noninferiority of LAA occlusion over warfarin for a composite endpoint of stroke, systemic embolism, and cardiovascular death,[23] there were methodological and safety concerns that led to regulators mandating a subsequent trial. Moreover, it has been suggested that the positive results from PROTECT AF may have resulted from issues with adjudication, favoring LAA occlusion, or a play of chance.[24] In the subsequent PREVAIL trial, LAA occlusion failed to meet its first coprimary efficacy endpoint of stroke, systemic embolism, and cardiovascular death and did not achieve the prespecified criteria for noninferiority compared with warfarin.[25] Troublingly, there were numerically more patients in the device arm who suffered from ischemic stroke compared with those who received warfarin,[25] which was subsequently confirmed in a patient-level meta-analysis of both the PROTECT AF and PREVAIL trials.[26] Taken together,

the results from these trials were far from conclusive in their support for LAA occlusion versus warfarin. Furthermore, there is a scarcity of data on the extended efficacy and safety of these lifelong devices, especially where the management of LAA leak and thrombus formation on occlusion devices are unclear.[27,28]

Pathophysiologically, although thromboembolism is believed to be the main mechanism of stroke in patients with AF, it is not the *only* mechanism. Therefore, although LAA occlusion may reduce embolic events originating from the LAA, it has no benefit in terms of protection against the hypercoagulable state in AF elsewhere.[1] Given our increased understanding of the multisystemic nature of AF, this approach in isolation may seem inadequate in comparison to "systemic" anticoagulation.

Over the years, the superiority of NOACs over warfarin has been cemented, as it has been shown to be comparable (or better) for stroke prevention with less major bleeding events, leading to its increasing use in a range of patients with AF.[16,29–31] As a result, it is important to bear in mind that there are other alternatives, apart from LAA occlusion, in patients who may be deemed unsuitable for anticoagulation with warfarin. In a prespecified analysis of the AVER-ROES trial, the investigators demonstrated that NOAC therapy with apixaban was tolerated in patients who previously failed treatment with warfarin due to poor anticoagulation control (42%), patient refusal (37%), and bleeding on vitamin K antagonist (8%).[32] The benefits of apixaban are confirmed in the long-term follow-up from this trial.[33] Moreover, for patients who are unable to tolerate even the shortest period of anticoagulation, the implantation of most LAA occlusion devices requires long-term antiplatelet therapy, which contributes to similar bleeding risks compared with OAC.[34,35]

In addition to the reasons stated earlier, there are other important considerations that guide the use of LAA occlusion as a last resort in AF. In many countries, most of the patients with AF are currently managed by primary care physicians who have had years of experience with the initiation and monitoring of OAC therapy. Consequently, extending the use of LAA occlusion to the general AF cohort according to patient choice will have a significant impact on the health care infrastructure by displacing the care of these patients to a few specialized centers that may be ill-equipped to deal with the influx of referrals and subsequent follow-up appointments; this is particularly true with the SARS-CoV 2019 pandemic, which is forcing many of us to reevaluate our delivery of health care to patients including the urgency and/or requirement for invasive procedures, including LAA occlusion[36]; this is partly driven by the increase in waiting lists due to limitations in terms of intensive care beds and anaesthesiology support and change in hospital workflows.

## LEFT ATRIAL APPENDAGE OCCLUSION FROM PATIENT CHOICE

From a patient perspective, it is important to highlight that there are other factors involved beyond mere efficacy and safety when ultimately deciding on the optimal treatment option. This includes long-term quality of life, overall satisfaction, and perceived inconvenience from potential side effects or complications. As part of our holistic care for these patients, it is therefore imperative to facilitate a shared decision-making process. In fact, this has been required for financial reimbursement of LAA occlusion in the United States, as per the Centers for Medicare & Medicaid Services.[37] In this setting, there is a case to respect patient autonomy, regardless of how *unwise* this decision may seem. Furthermore, the chance to avoid anticoagulation as afforded by LAA occlusion may be desired by certain patients according to lifestyle preferences (eg, participation in high-risk contact sports). Several shared decision-making tools have previously been evaluated for stroke prevention in AF, although their role in LAA occlusion remains to be determined.[38]

In terms of stroke prevention for AF, although the need for alternative treatment options is greatest among patients with contraindications to OAC, there is a paradox in that the LAA occlusion trials were not conducted for this purpose by strictly excluding patients who were deemed ineligible for anticoagulation.[23,25] Instead, these trials were essentially conducted to investigate whether LAA occlusion may be used as an alternative first-line option in patients with AF. Although we have discussed the limitations of these trials earlier, it certainly does not disregard them as viable alternatives. Moreover, there are good observational real-world data to support the use of LAA occlusion in patients beyond that, which were studied in the randomized controlled trials.[16–18,39,40]

It is also important to consider that some patients may decide to undergo endo-epicardial LAA occlusion with an LARIAT device (Sentre-HEART, Redwood City, CA, USA), despite an excess risk of major procedural complications,[41,42] as the lack of foreign body within the endocardial surface of the left atrium removes the need for any form of long-term antithrombotic therapy. In this regard, patients may be willing to be exposed to a greater initial risk if this is balanced by an improvement in quality of life and subsequent reduction in bleeding events. Furthermore, patients may have high levels of anxiety poststroke,[43] especially in those with AF who were already on anticoagulation therapy before these events and are discharged on the same treatment. In such patients with resistant stroke, there may be a role for LAA occlusion,[44] and even combination therapy for LAA occlusion and OAC,[45,46] although this warrants further investigation.

Although direct head-to-head comparisons of LAA occlusion versus NOAC are lacking, network meta-analyses in this area have suggested that LAA occlusion may be superior to NOAC in terms of reduction of major bleeding but associated with increased ischemic events.[47,48] The PRAGUE-17 trial is the only prospective randomized controlled trial that has compared LAA occlusion against NOAC therapy, and it found no significant difference in the annual rates of the composite outcome of stroke, transient ischemic attack, systemic embolism, cardiovascular death, major or nonmajor clinically relevant bleeding, or procedure-/device-related complications among patients with AF with a high-risk of stroke and bleeding.[49] These findings were corroborated by a recent study of patients enrolled in the Amulet Observational Registry, where LAA occlusion was reported to have similar efficacy for stroke prevention but lower risk of major bleeding and all-cause mortality compared with propensity score–matched controls with AF who were treated with NOACs from the Danish national patient registries.[50] Arguments supporting the use of LAA based on patient choice or as a last resort in patients with AF are summarized in **Fig. 1**.

## HOW TO APPROACH THE PATIENT

As clinicians, we should be equipped with an in-depth understanding of the most current data on LAA occlusion and its limitations and be prepared to discuss this as treatment option with patients, where it may be appropriate. The appropriateness for LAA occlusion often largely depends on the constraints of our health care systems including the availability of local resources. For publicly funded systems (eg, the National Health Service in the United Kingdom), cost-effectiveness may be paramount, whereas in privately owned systems (eg, in the United States), patient choice may have a bigger impact

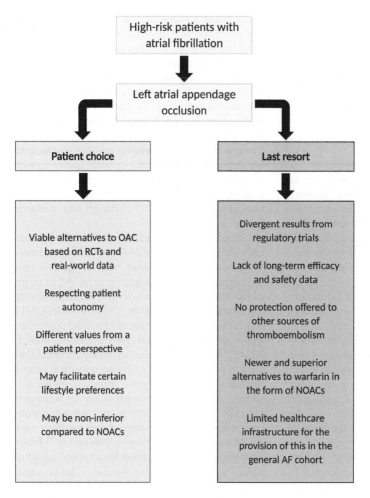

**Fig. 1.** Arguments supporting the use of left atrial appendage based on patient choice or as a last resort in patients with atrial fibrillation. AF, atrial fibrillation; NOAC, nonvitamin K oral antagonist; OAC, oral anticoagulation; RCT, randomized controlled trial.

on the chosen treatment. Compared with OAC, LAA occlusion is associated with a higher upfront cost that eventually balances out after about 10 years with greater cost-effectiveness beyond this period.[51–53] For this reason, our discussion with patients should incorporate at least a 5-year horizon (and possibly a 10-year horizon), as it also ensures that the upfront risk from the procedure is counterbalanced by the long-term benefit (Supplementary Materials). It may be helpful to break the preprocedural discussion into 2 parts: "whether-to" and "how-to." The "whether-to" discussion may be led by nonimplanting or referring physicians, as it encompasses a general discussion surrounding the benefits and potential risks of the procedure, considering the patients views and perspectives; this may be supplemented with a multidisciplinary team approach. Once a preliminary decision has been made to proceed with LAA occlusion, then a further discussion on "how-to" can be led by the implanting physician.

It should be highlighted that the following section is based on our opinion of how to approach patients in terms of LAA occlusion. In a setting where there is limited provision for LAA occlusion, we propose that it should first be reserved for high-risk patients with AF ($CHA_2DS_2$-VASc score of $\geq 2$ in men and $\geq 3$ in women) who have an absolute contraindication to and no other requirement for long-term anticoagulation. Although there are no prospective randomized controlled trials in this specific group of patients, it is clear that they have greatest clinical need for LAA occlusion and that nontreatment exposes them to a significant risk of thromboembolic complications. Nonetheless, it is important to consider whether these absolute contraindications are fixed and/or permanent. For example, although patients who in the third trimester of pregnancy may be unsuitable for OAC, this is a temporary state. In contrast, patients with inheritable bleeding disorders have a fixed and likely permanent condition. Furthermore, it is important to review and optimize the management of these other conditions (eg, surgery), where possible.

If there is excess capacity to perform LAA occlusion, it may be considered for patients with AF with relative contraindications to anticoagulation, resistant stroke, poor quality of anticoagulation control, drug-drug interactions, or severe side effects to OAC. Among patients with relative contraindications to OAC due to a high-risk of bleeding, every attempt to manage the bleeding risk factors should be made in the first instance. For patients with an unacceptably high risk of bleeding despite this, LAA occlusion may be considered, provided they are able to tolerate a period of enhanced antithrombotic treatment followed by lifelong antiplatelet therapy. Patients with resistant stroke while prescribed OAC should have a review of their compliance to therapy. In those with resistant stroke despite good adherence to OAC, an alternative OAC agent should be used instead in the long-term or LAA occlusion may be considered. If these patients have a second recurrence despite an alternative OAC agent, then LAA occlusion should be considered. Patients on warfarin who have a poor quality of anticoagulation control should be switched to a NOAC. Poor compliance to treatment should, in our opinion, not be considered as an isolated reason for LAA occlusion, as there remains a requirement for patient compliance with drug therapy post-device implantation. Drug-drug interactions and severe side effects can often be managed by using an alternative OAC agent (or by changing the other offending drug in the case of drug-drug interactions). In patients who have severe drug-drug interactions despite multiple trials, LAA occlusion may be appropriate.

Of note, patient frailty is a very important consideration and a potential reason for recommending against LAA occlusion even in the presence of a strong contraindication to OAC. There are 2 main reasons for this. First, LAA occlusion is associated with up to a 1 in 100 risks of device embolization or cardiac tamponade, sometimes requiring emergency open surgery, which frail patients may be less likely to survive. Second, the long-term survival of patients is strongly

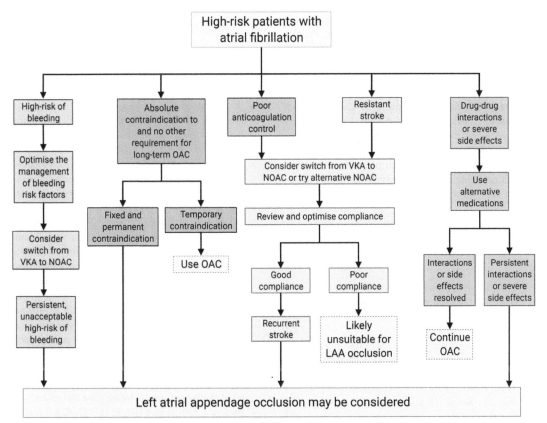

**Fig. 2.** Algorithm for the selection of high-risk patients with atrial fibrillation for left atrial appendage occlusion. LAA, left atrial appendage; NOAC, non-vitamin K antagonist oral anticoagulant; OAC, oral anticoagulant; VKA, vitamin K antagonist.

related to their baseline frailty status, and for this reason LAA occlusion has been restricted to patients with a Rockwood clinical frailty score of 6 or less.[54] Increasingly, and perhaps not surprisingly, many patients referred for LAA occlusion are seen to be suffering from dementia; this makes informed discussions with patients challenging, and so it is always important to involve family members into the decision-making process. We should also have a low threshold for requesting a formal neurologic assessment for dementia if there are any uncertainties.

We acknowledge we have presented a nonexhaustive list of scenarios that may be encountered in clinical practice (**Fig. 2**). However, we hope that the principles discussed here can be applied to other situations as a guide for clinicians in their selection of patients for LAA occlusion. Presently, we do not believe that there is sufficient evidence to offer LAA occlusion as first-line treatment of stroke prevention in AF on the sole basis of patient choice alone.

## SUMMARY

LAA occlusion may be a viable alternative to OAC for high-risk patients with AF. However, patient selection remains an important aspect of treatment, and further studies are required to demonstrate the role of LAA occlusion compared with OAC in specific subgroups. An individualized and multidisciplinary team approach should be adopted in patients who are being considered for LAA occlusion, especially with the current paradigm of comprehensively characterizing and evaluating patients with AF[55] and managing such patients in an integrated or holistic manner, which has been associated with improved clinical outcomes.[56,57]

## CLINICS CARE POINTS

- LAA occlusion may be noninferior to OAC in high-risk patients with AF without contraindications to long-term anticoagulation.

- The efficacy and safety of LAA occlusion remains unproved in patients with absolute contraindications to OAC and other subgroups.

- Patient choice is an important consideration but current data do not support it to be the predominant reason for the choice of LAA occlusion over OAC.

## DISCLOSURE

W.Y. Ding: none declared. G.Y.H. Lip: consultant and speaker for BMS/Pfizer, Boehringer Ingelheim, and Daiichi-Sankyo. No fees are directly received personally. D. Gupta: Speaker for Boehringer Ingelheim, Biosense Webster, and Boston Scientific; Proctor for Abbott. Research Grants from Medtronic, Biosense Webster, and Boston Scientific. All authors declare no conflict of interest.

## SUPPLEMENTARY DATA

Supplementary data related to this article can be found online at https://doi.org/10.1016/j.iccl.2021.11.006.

## REFERENCES

1. Ding WY, Gupta D, Lip GYH. Atrial fibrillation and the prothrombotic state: revisiting Virchow's triad in 2020. Heart 2020;106:1463–8.
2. Hindricks G, Potpara T, Dagres N, et al. 2020 ESC Guidelines for the diagnosis and management of atrial fibrillation developed in collaboration with the European Association of Cardio-Thoracic Surgery (EACTS). Eur Heart J 2021;42:373–498.
3. January CT, Wann LS, Alpert JS, et al. 2014 AHA/ACC/HRS guideline for the management of patients with atrial fibrillation: executive summary: a report of the American College of Cardiology/American Heart Association Task Force on practice guidelines and the Heart Rhythm Society. Circulation 2014;130:2071–104.
4. Lip GYH, Banerjee A, Boriani G, et al. Antithrombotic therapy for atrial fibrillation: CHEST guideline and expert panel report. Chest 2018;154:1121–201.
5. Verma A, Cairns JA, Mitchell LB, et al. 2014 focused update of the Canadian Cardiovascular Society Guidelines for the management of atrial fibrillation. Can J Cardiol 2014;30:1114–30.
6. O'Brien EC, Holmes DN, Ansell JE, et al. Physician practices regarding contraindications to oral anticoagulation in atrial fibrillation: findings from the outcomes registry for better informed treatment of atrial fibrillation (ORBIT-AF) registry. Am Heart J 2014;167:601–9.e1.
7. Steinberg BA, Greiner MA, Hammill BG, et al. Contraindications to anticoagulation therapy and eligibility for novel anticoagulants in older patients with atrial fibrillation. Cardiovasc Ther 2015;33:177–83.
8. Kachroo S, Hamilton M, Liu X, et al. Oral anticoagulant discontinuation in patients with nonvalvular atrial fibrillation. Am J Manag Care 2016;22:e1–8.
9. Hwang J, Han S, Bae H-J, et al. NOAC adherence of patients with atrial fibrillation in the real world: dosing frequency matters? Thromb Haemost 2020;120:306–13.

10. Proietti M, Lane DA. The compelling issue of non-vitamin K antagonist oral anticoagulant adherence in atrial fibrillation patients: a systematic need for new strategies. Thromb Haemost 2020;120:369–71.

11. Kakkar AK, Mueller I, Bassand J-P, et al. Risk profiles and antithrombotic treatment of patients newly diagnosed with atrial fibrillation at risk of stroke: perspectives from the international, observational, prospective GARFIELD registry. PLoS One 2013;8:e63479.

12. Pritchett RV, Bem D, Turner GM, et al. Improving the prescription of oral anticoagulants in atrial fibrillation: a systematic review. Thromb Haemost 2019;119:294–307.

13. Aberg H. Atrial fibrillation. I. A study of atrial thrombosis and systemic embolism in a necropsy material. Acta Med Scand 1969;185:373–9.

14. Blackshear JL, Odell JA. Appendage obliteration to reduce stroke in cardiac surgical patients with atrial fibrillation. Ann Thorac Surg 1996;61:755–9.

15. Mahajan R, Brooks AG, Sullivan T, et al. Importance of the underlying substrate in determining thrombus location in atrial fibrillation: implications for left atrial appendage closure. Heart 2012;98:1120–6.

16. Enomoto Y, Gadiyaram VK, Gianni C, et al. Use of non-warfarin oral anticoagulants instead of warfarin during left atrial appendage closure with the Watchman device. Hear Rhythm 2017;14:19–24.

17. Boersma LV, Ince H, Kische S, et al. Evaluating real-world clinical outcomes in atrial fibrillation patients receiving the WATCHMAN left atrial appendage closure technology. Circ Arrhythm Electrophysiol 2019;12:e006841.

18. Ding WY, Lip GYH, Bartoletti S, et al. Long-term outcomes of left atrial appendage occlusion in high-risk atrial fibrillation patients: 4-year follow up data. J Thromb Thrombolysis 2021;51:1090–3.

19. Glikson M, Wolff R, Hindricks G, et al. EHRA/EAPCI expert consensus statement on catheter-based left atrial appendage occlusion - an update. Europace 2019;15:1133–80.

20. Piccini JP, Sievert H, Patel MR. Left atrial appendage occlusion: rationale, evidence, devices, and patient selection. Eur Heart J 2017;38:869–76.

21. Munir MB, Khan MZ, Darden D, et al. Contemporary procedural trends of Watchman percutaneous left atrial appendage occlusion in the United States. *J Cardiovasc Electrophysiol* Published Online First: 2020. https://doi.org/10.1111/jce.14804.

22. January CT, Wann LS, Calkins H, et al. 2019 AHA/ACC/HRS Focused Update of the 2014 AHA/ACC/HRS Guideline for the Management of Patients With Atrial Fibrillation: A Report of the American College of Cardiology/American Heart Association Task Force on Clinical Practice Guidelines and the Heart R. J Am Coll Cardiol 2019;74:104–32.

23. Holmes DR, Reddy VY, Turi ZG, et al. Percutaneous closure of the left atrial appendage versus warfarin therapy for prevention of stroke in patients with atrial fibrillation: a randomised non-inferiority trial. Lancet 2009;374:534–42.

24. Mandrola J, Foy A, Naccarelli G. Percutaneous left atrial appendage closure is not ready for routine clinical use. Hear Rhythm 2018;15:298–301.

25. Holmes DRJ, Kar S, Price MJ, et al. Prospective randomized evaluation of the Watchman Left Atrial Appendage Closure device in patients with atrial fibrillation versus long-term warfarin therapy: the PREVAIL trial. J Am Coll Cardiol 2014;64:1–12.

26. Holmes DRJ, Doshi SK, Kar S, et al. Left atrial appendage closure as an alternative to warfarin for stroke prevention in atrial fibrillation: a patient-level meta-analysis. J Am Coll Cardiol 2015;65:2614–23.

27. Fauchier L, Cinaud A, Brigadeau F, et al. Device-related thrombosis after percutaneous left atrial appendage occlusion for atrial fibrillation. J Am Coll Cardiol 2018;71:1528–36.

28. Dukkipati SR, Kar S, Holmes DR, et al. Device-related thrombus after left atrial appendage closure: incidence, predictors, and outcomes. Circulation 2018;138:874–85.

29. Cavallari I, Verolino G, Romano S, et al. Efficacy and safety of nonvitamin k oral anticoagulants in patients with atrial fibrillation and cancer: a study-level meta-analysis. Thromb Haemost 2020;120:314–21.

30. Hohnloser SH, Basic E, Nabauer M. Changes in oral anticoagulation therapy over one year in 51,000 atrial fibrillation patients at risk for stroke: a practice-derived study. Thromb Haemost 2019;119:882–93.

31. Hohmann C, Hohnloser SH, Jacob J, et al. Non-Vitamin K oral anticoagulants in comparison to phenprocoumon in geriatric and non-geriatric patients with non-valvular atrial fibrillation. Thromb Haemost 2019;119:971–80.

32. Coppens M, Synhorst D, Eikelboom JW, et al. Efficacy and safety of apixaban compared with aspirin in patients who previously tried but failed treatment with vitamin K antagonists: results from the AVERROES trial. Eur Heart J 2014;35:1856–63.

33. Benz AP, Eikelboom JW, Yusuf S, et al. Long-Term Treatment with Apixaban in Patients with Atrial Fibrillation: Outcomes during the Open-Label Extension following AVERROES. Thromb Haemost 2021;121:518–28.

34. Diener H-C, Eikelboom J, Connolly SJ, et al. Apixaban versus aspirin in patients with atrial fibrillation and previous stroke or transient ischaemic attack: a predefined subgroup analysis from AVERROES, a randomised trial. Lancet Neurol 2012;11:225–31.

35. Connolly SJ, Eikelboom J, Joyner C, et al. Apixaban in patients with atrial fibrillation. N Engl J Med 2011;364:806–17.

36. Freixa X, Aminian A, De Backer O, et al. Left atrial appendage occlusion in COVID-19 times. Eur Hear J Suppl 2020;22:P47–52.

37. Jensen TS, Chin J, Ashb L, et al. Decision Memo for Percutaneous Left Atrial Appendage (LAA) Closure Therapy (CAG-00445N). 2016. Available at: https://www.cms.gov/medicare-coverage-database/details/nca-decision-memo.aspx?NCAId=281.

38. Torres Roldan VD, Brand-McCarthy SR, Ponce OJ, et al. Shared decision making tools for people facing stroke prevention strategies in atrial fibrillation: a systematic review and environmental scan. Med Decis Mak 2021;41:540–9.

39. Freeman JV, Varosy P, Price MJ, et al. The NCDR left atrial appendage occlusion registry. J Am Coll Cardiol 2020;75:1503–18.

40. Reddy VY, Mobius-Winkler S, Miller MA, et al. Left atrial appendage closure with the Watchman device in patients with a contraindication for oral anticoagulation: the ASAP study (ASA Plavix Feasibility Study With Watchman Left Atrial Appendage Closure Technology). J Am Coll Cardiol 2013;61:2551–6.

41. Price MJ, Gibson DN, Yakubov SJ, et al. Early safety and efficacy of percutaneous left atrial appendage suture ligation: results from the U.S. transcatheter LAA ligation consortium. J Am Coll Cardiol 2014;64:565–72.

42. US Food and Drug Administration. Lariat Suture Delivery Device for Left Atrial Appendage (LAA) Closure by SentreHEART: FDA Safety Communication - Reports of Patient Deaths and Other Serious Adverse Events. Available at: https://wayback.archive-it.org/7993/20170112164108/http://www.fda.gov/Safety/MedWatch/SafetyInformation/SafetyAlertsforHumanMedicalProducts/ucm454660.htm. Accessed Feburary 17, 2021.

43. Kapoor A, Si K, Yu AYX, et al. Younger age and depressive symptoms predict high risk of generalized anxiety after stroke and transient ischemic attack. Stroke 2019;50:2359–63.

44. Cruz-González I, González-Ferreiro R, Freixa X, et al. Left atrial appendage occlusion for stroke despite oral anticoagulation (resistant stroke). Results from the Amplatzer Cardiac Plug registry. Rev Esp Cardiol 2020;73:28–34.

45. Masjuan J, Salido L, DeFelipe A, et al. Oral anticoagulation and left atrial appendage closure: a new strategy for recurrent cardioembolic stroke. Eur J Neurol 2019;26:816–20.

46. Freixa X, Cruz-González I, Regueiro A, et al. Left atrial appendage occlusion as adjunctive therapy to anticoagulation for stroke recurrence. J Invasive Cardiol 2019;31:212–6.

47. Li X, Wen S-N, Li S-N, et al. Over 1-year efficacy and safety of left atrial appendage occlusion versus novel oral anticoagulants for stroke prevention in atrial fibrillation: A systematic review and meta-analysis of randomized controlled trials and observational studies. Hear Rhythm 2016;13:1203–14.

48. Koifman E, Lipinski MJ, Escarcega RO, et al. Comparison of Watchman device with new oral anticoagulants in patients with atrial fibrillation: A network meta-analysis. Int J Cardiol 2016;205:17–22.

49. Osmancik P, Herman D, Neuzil P, et al. Left atrial appendage closure versus direct oral anticoagulants in high-risk patients with atrial fibrillation. J Am Coll Cardiol 2020;75:3122–35.

50. Nielsen-Kudsk JE, Korsholm K, Damgaard D, et al. Clinical outcomes associated with left atrial appendage occlusion versus direct oral anticoagulation in atrial fibrillation. JACC Cardiovasc Interv 2021;14:69–78.

51. Panikker S, Lord J, Jarman JWE, et al. Outcomes and costs of left atrial appendage closure from randomized controlled trial and real-world experience relative to oral anticoagulation. Eur Heart J 2016;37:3470–82.

52. Reddy VY, Akehurst RL, Gavaghan MB, et al. Cost-effectiveness of left atrial appendage closure for stroke reduction in atrial fibrillation: analysis of pooled, 5-year, long-term data. J Am Heart Assoc 2019;8:e011577.

53. Reddy VY, Akehurst RL, Amorosi SL, et al. Cost-effectiveness of left atrial appendage closure with the WATCHMAN device compared with warfarin or non-vitamin k antagonist oral anticoagulants for secondary prevention in nonvalvular atrial fibrillation. Stroke 2018;49:1464–70.

54. Ding WY, Gupta D. Percutaneous left atrial appendage occlusion: a view from the UK. Arrhythmia Electrophysiol Rev 2020;9:83–7.

55. Potpara TS, Lip GYH, Blomstrom-Lundqvist C, et al. The 4S-AF Scheme (Stroke Risk; Symptoms; Severity of Burden; Substrate): a novel approach to in-depth characterization (rather than classification) of atrial fibrillation. Thromb Haemost 2020. https://doi.org/10.1055/s-0040-1716408.

56. Lip GYH. The ABC pathway: an integrated approach to improve AF management. Nat Rev Cardiol 2017;14:627–8.

57. Yoon M, Yang P-S, Jang E, et al. Improved population-based clinical outcomes of patients with atrial fibrillation by compliance with the simple ABC (atrial fibrillation better care) pathway for integrated care management: A Nationwide Cohort Study. Thromb Haemost 2019;119:1695–703.

# Pre-cath Laboratory Planning for Left Atrial Appendage Occlusion – Optional or Essential?

Jasneet Devgun, DO[a], Tom De Potter, MD[b],
Davide Fabbricatore, MD[b], Dee Dee Wang, MD[a,*]

## KEYWORDS

- Left atrial appendage occlusion • Left atrial appendage • Atrial fibrillation • Cardiac CT
- 3D printing • Imaging • Structural heart disease

## KEY POINTS

- Left atrial appendage occlusion for atrial fibrillation comes with risks of complications such as improper device sizing with consequent device leak, device embolization, or cardiac injury
- Two-dimensional imaging technologies provide an incomplete understanding of the complexity of the left atrial appendage anatomy
- Preprocedural planning for left atrial appendage occlusion with cardiac CT is shown to increase procedural accuracy
- Further benefits can be achieved with 3D printing, computational modeling, artificial intelligence, as well as intraprocedural 3D angiography and dynamic fusion imaging

## INTRODUCTION

Over the course of the last 2 decades, transcatheter structural interventions have experienced exponential growth and rapid evolution driven by near-Promethean innovation and multidisciplinary biomedical ingenuity. In the wake of this development, the need for multimodality imaging for structural heart procedures has been recognized as an important and arguably essential adjunct used in all phases of the procedural process. From preprocedural planning and teaching to guidance within the cath lab, as well as to postprocedural care, structural imaging is proving to be an indispensable asset to ensuring procedural success. Given the inherent complexity of cardiac anatomy, an in-depth understanding of anatomy and physiology is vital for the success of structural heart procedures.

Structural imaging has established its utility in procedures such as transcatheter aortic valve replacement (TAVR), mitral valve interventions such as transcatheter mitral valve replacement (TMVR) and MitraClip (Abbott, Illinois, USA), as well as septal defect repairs. For left atrial appendage occlusion (LAAO), multi-modality imaging is gaining traction and is, likewise, arguably essential in all phases of procedural planning and execution. In the setting of a global pandemic with limited access to personal protection equipment for health care providers, maximizing the efficiency and safety of delivery of health care using modernized imaging

[a] Division of Cardiology, Henry Ford Health System, 2799 West Grand Boulevard, Clara Ford Pavilion, Detroit, MI 48202, USA; [b] Cardiovascular Center, Onze-Lieve-Vrouwziekenhuis Hospital, Moorselbaan 164, Aalst 9300, Belgium
* Corresponding author.
E-mail address: dwang2@hfhs.org

Intervent Cardiol Clin 11 (2022) 143–152
https://doi.org/10.1016/j.iccl.2021.11.003
2211-7458/22/© 2021 Elsevier Inc. All rights reserved.

technologies has become even more critical. Our review of the literature seeks to synthesize the critical thinking methodologies to investing time in planning for LAAO procedures.

## PERCUTANEOUS LEFT ATRIAL APPENDAGE OCCLUSION

### Understanding the Rationale for Periprocedural Evaluation

Common terminology of the left atrial appendage anatomy assumes the orifice of the LAAO landing zone is a circle. With this assumption, 2D transesophageal echocardiogram (TEE) imaging was instituted as the gold standard of imaging the LAA for sizing and device selection. Optimal viewing angles were depicted as 0, 45, 90, and 135°. However, the arrival of multi-detector CT has demonstrated the LAA's landing zone to be elliptical and at times amorphous in shape with multiple angulations that are unique to each patient's anatomy. Traditional 2D TEE and the narrow imaging field of 2D intra-cardiac echo (ICE) are unable to visualize the full dimensions of the LAA due to the inability of operators to obtain coaxiality to the true maximal dimensions of the LAA. Hence, modern day LAAO implantation outcomes in the published literature have not achieved 100% procedural success rates. Increasing procedural success and safety outcomes of LAAO technologies requires an in-depth preoperative understanding of each patient's unique LAA anatomy.

### Procedure details

In the United States, the WATCHMAN (Boston Scientific, Marlborough, Massachusetts), WATCHMAN FLX (Boston Scientific, Marlborough, Massachusetts) and Amulet (Abbott, Abbott Park, Illinois) have received approval by the Food and Drug Administration for the prevention of stroke in patients with atrial fibrillation (AF).[1] The FLX and the Amulet LAAO devices are seated in the LAA, the most common site of intracardiac thrombus formation in AF, to prevent thrombi from forming within it thereby preventing cardio-embolic phenomenon.[2–4] Due to timing of FDA regulatory approval, currently, the most widely studied LAAO devices in the United States are the WATCHMAN and WATCHMAN FLX LAAO systems. Hence, subsequent procedural details will focus on WATCHMAN FLX delivery systems.

The WATCHMAN FLX LAAO procedure itself begins with obtaining femoral venous access. Transseptal puncture is performed, usually under TEE guidance, to enter into the left atrium (Fig. 1). The optimal transseptal puncture site assessed by TEE is often limited by the fact that we are obtaining 2D images of a 3D structure. Assessing whether one is puncturing too anterior or posterior in the septal plane is difficult. Furthermore, the generation of 3D images, although possible, is limited by the quality of the initial 2D images obtained, which may not render a very precise assessment and execution of this maneuver.

Once transseptal puncture is performed, a guidewire is sent to the left atrium and into the left superior pulmonary vein. The WATCHMAN or WATCHMAN FLX access sheath and dilator are advanced over the guidewire into the left atrium. Dilator and guidewire are removed followed by the advancement of the angled pigtail catheter through the WATCHMAN access sheath into the distal portion of the main lobe of the LAA for the contrast visualization of the LAA.[5] Next, the access sheath is advanced into the LAA over the pigtail catheter until the access sheath radiopaque marker band meets the corresponding device size marker band or is just distal to the LAA ostium. Once identified, the pigtail catheter is removed, and the LAA occluder delivery system is advanced through the access sheath. Under fluoroscopic guidance, the delivery system's distal marker band is aligned to the distal marker of the access sheath.[5] Traditionally, confirmation of delivery sheath positioning and coaxiality is verified by TEE. Both fluoroscopic and TEE verification of coaxiality are primarily by 2D images that, by nature, confer an incomplete overall visualization of the LAA ostium and optimal coaxial positioning, which may lead to incomplete seating of the LAA occlude, device leaks, among other complications.

The WATCHMAN FLX device is then deployed into the LAA via a combination of passive exposure and advancement of the FLX ball, consisting of retracting the access sheath and delivery system while stabilizing the deployment knob. After the deployment of the device, positioning is evaluated under TEE guidance and contrast fluoroscopy. Specific criteria of appropriate positioning must be met, which includes position, anchor, size, and seal (PASS). Ideally, the LAA occluder would be placed at the level of the circumflex artery with minimal protrusion into the left atrium. A "tug test" is then performed, for which the deployment knob is pulled and the LAAO device is visualized under fluoroscopy, confirming adequate anchoring of the device. Device compression should be at a minimum of 8%, and peridevice flow should be no more than 5 mm at vena contracta on 2D TEE color flow.

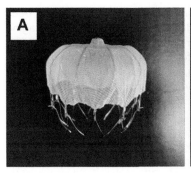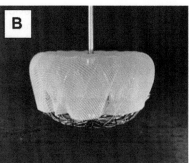

Fig. 1. The WATCHMAN (*A*) and WATCHMAN FLX (*B*) devices. The original WATCHMAN is a self-expanding nitinol structure with a porous polyethylene terephthalate (PET) membrane on the proximal face. The WATCHMAN FLX is a modified version with the rearrangement of the nitinol structure at the distal end into a rounded configuration and extension of the PET membrane distally.

## Pre-cath Laboratory Planning in Left Atrial Appendage Occlusion

Traditionally, two-dimensional TEE had been the sole imaging modality to guide LAAO procedures until 2011, when computed tomography (CT) began being integrated into cath laboratory planning and postprocedure monitoring.[6] While CT had become standard of care for transcatheter device planning, such as for TAVR and transcatheter mitral replacement therapies, it had not been in use for LAAO until recently.[7,8]

Stand-alone fluoroscopic sizing for LAA in the cardiac catheterization or electrophysiology laboratory without preprocedural imaging has several limitations. Contrast injection with fluoroscopic evaluation in multiple c-arm angle projections provides an overview of the shape of the LAA but is unable to verify maximal coaxial alignment to the true orifice of the LAA landing zone. Off-axis fluoroscopic projections of the LAA may lead to under or oversizing of the LAA landing zone, and the inability to appreciate challenging anatomy. Hence, in patients without access to intraprocedural TEE or preprocedural CT imaging planning, pure fluoroscopic guidance has a lower device implantation success rate than with standard of care TEE imaging guidance. This may result in aborted LAAO procedures due to inappropriate anatomy for the devices available, or LAA anatomy that may not have been compatible with any commercially available device.

However, TEE for LAA closure, although an additive value to fluoroscopic imaging alone, itself also has inherent limitations. Patients undergoing outpatient TEE are usually volume depleted due to necessary fasting nothing by mouth requirements before the procedure. As the LAA volume depends on loading conditions, TEE can certainly underestimate the LAA dimensions.[9] Also, the spatial resolution of TEE is limited and somewhat operator- and image quality dependent, which may lead to the underappreciation of LAA contractility and dimensions changes during the cardiac cycle.[10]

Furthermore, in the setting of the 2019 global SARS-CoV-2 pandemic, access to outpatient preprocedural TEE became a barrier to scheduling patients for LAAO procedures. Given the inherent risks of aerosolization procedures and spread of SARS-CoV-2 coupled with a limited global supply of personal protection equipment, echocardiography laboratories across the world decreased their elective TEE procedural volume to ration the supply of personal protection equipment.[11,12] In some countries, once the supply of personal protection equipment for health care providers became more readily available, mandatory nasopharyngeal swab testing for COVID-19 before any preprocedural TEE became a secondary deterrent for patient's seeking access to LAAO procedures. Hence, a migration away from preprocedural TEE has been accelerated by the global pandemic into alternative additive technologies to support intraprocedural case guidance.

### Planning Modalities

Left atrial appendage occlusion is a procedure that has the potential to attain immense gains from not only the integration of CT but also of other imaging modalities as well such as 3D printing, computational modeling (CM), and artificial intelligence (AI).

### *Computed Tomography*

Preprocedural planning for LAAO now consists not only of TEE imaging but also multidetector ECG-gated, contrast-enhanced cardiac CT. Modern advanced dual-source cardiac CT scanners allow for adequate image acquisition and evaluation of patients with irregular heart rates due to post-scan additive features such as EKG editing.[13] The benefits of CT imaging before LAAO are manifold, ranging from the assessment of patient appropriateness (eg, congenitally-absent LAA, prior surgical or transcatheter device, or the presence of LAA thrombus), to the structural characterization of the LAA itself, as well as accurate sizing of the device and localization of the appropriate landing zones of the LAA occluder with precision (Fig. 2). Furthermore, CT images can be further processed to form 3D print models, which can offer substantial preprocedural planning.

### 3D printing

Three-dimensional printing is a method of manufacturing three-dimensional physical objects from information derived from digital media (Fig. 3).[14] The process of forming three-dimensional physical objects starts with obtaining high-quality imaging data and its conversion to a Digital Imaging and Communication in Medicine (DICOM) format for further image processing. Processing is done through special software to define and build the anatomic body parts of interest in a process called *segmentation*. Subsequently, 3D volume rendering and digital modeling of patient-specific anatomy are constructed. Patient-specific 3D digital anatomic models are then saved in a stereolithography (STL) file format, which contains the surface mesh information of the specific geometries to be used in the 3D printing process, which can be further refined by computer-aided design modeling and computational analysis. Finally, a 3D print model is made by processing and using this digital information to create physical objects by depositing multiple layers of material over digitally defined geometries.

Three-dimensional print models have demonstrated that patient anatomy is much more complex than what is understood by traditional two dimensional TEE imaging alone (Fig. 4).[14,15] The clinical implications of this is that our knowledge of LAAO device sizing as well as identifying appropriate landing zone and deployment, is far more primitive than what

was previously understood, as may have been our clinical decisions using traditional imaging methods. Three-dimensional printing has great implications for improving procedural accuracy, device sizing, and time to reaching the early operator learning curve, among many other benefits.[7,14,15]

### Intraprocedural 3D angiography

Rotational angiography or 3D angiography is an imaging modality that allows intraprocedural reconstruction of a 3D model of a chamber of interest such as the LA (including the LAA), yielding datasets much like those derived from cardiac CT. Images can be overlaid on 2D fluoroscopy for anatomic guidance and can be used for LAA sizing and device selection as an alternative to TEE. As the images are acquired on the same table using the same equipment as the 2D fluoroscopy, they can be used to visualize the ideal angulation of the fluoroscopy tube for a particular LAA, eliminating issues of foreshortening.[16] As these images are obtained by contrast injection during apnea and rapid ventricular pacing, a workflow using general anesthesia is typically required for obtaining good image quality.

### Dynamic fusion imaging

In day-to-day practice, physicians performing LAA closure have to be able to synthesize and recreate the images obtained by different imaging modalities and techniques into one 3D understanding of the LAA in their mind. However, when initial image acquisition is only performed with 2D TEE or fluoroscopic datasets, a full understanding of the LAA may not be possible. Currently, pre-procedural CT generated LAA caseplans are not able to be fused onto fluoroscopic displays. Hence, the role of dynamic fusion imaging in LAAO is gaining greater interest in the transcatheter arena.

The dynamic fusion imaging technique has the ability to merge the information obtained from different methods onto one fluoroscopic display.

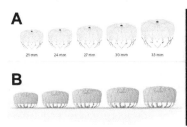
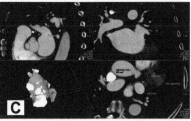

Fig. 2. (A) The WATCHMAN device is produced in various sizes, as shown above. (B) The WATCHMAN FLX comes in the following sizes from left to right: 20 mm, 24 mm, 27 mm, 31 mm, and 35 mm. (C) CT-guided LAA sizing to aid in choosing the appropriate device size. (Images from Boston Scientific. ©

2021 Boston Scientific Corporation or its affiliates. All rights reserved.)

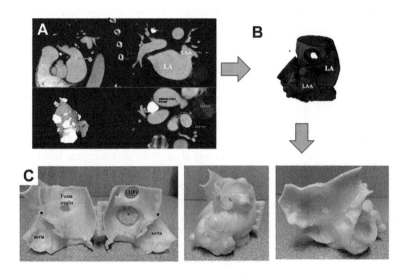

**Fig. 3.** The process of LAA image acquisition and processing is displayed in this figure. (*A*) A series of frames was taken during CT imaging for visualizing the appendage and its landing zone with accurate measuring of the maximum and minimum diameter, LAA orifice area, and length of LAA from the landing zone. The CT images are processed via 3D volume-rendering into a digital format and structure (*B*), which in turn can be used to create 3D print models (*C*) for a more in-depth understanding of LAA anatomy and for the use of preprocedural simulation. The 3D model demonstrates the fossa ovalis (bottom left & bottom right, labeled as FO) between the SVC and IVC, demonstrating optimal transseptal puncture site. The WATCHMAN device is seen well-seated in the LAA orifice. FO: fossa ovalis, IVC: inferior vena cava, LA: left atrium, LAA: left atrial appendage, SVC: superior vena cava.

Specifically, for LAA closure, anatomic landmarks identified by TEE or CT are directly overlaid on the real-time fluoroscopy, the latter typically being superior for identifying the closure device itself. Thus, these systems aim to generate a single final real-time hybrid visualization of the aforementioned techniques, improving safety and reducing procedural times. Several vendors offer integrated TEE/fluoroscopy or 3DRA/fluoroscopy modalities (**Fig. 5**).[17–20]

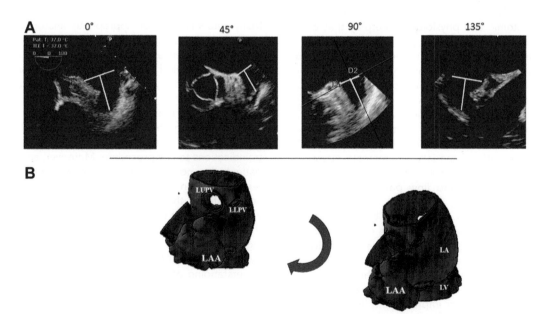

**Fig. 4.** Images of left atrial appendage taken by TEE in various standard views to take measurements of the appendage (*A*). As seen from left to right, these views are taken approximately at 0, 45, 90, and 135°. Transesophageal echocardiography gives us an incomplete understanding of the true complex nature of LAA anatomy (*B*). These are 3D images of the left atrium and LAA taken from the same patient's CT scan images. One can see the complex entry point and curved direction the appendage takes, which would have significant implications on device sizing and deployment. LA: left atrium, LAA: left atrial appendage, LLPV: left lower pulmonary vein, LUPV: left upper pulmonary vein.

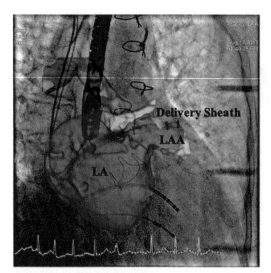

Fig. 5. This figure shows a 3D model of the LA, partially cut-away. A Watchman delivery sheath with a loaded Watchman device is positioned in the LAA and is ready for deployment. LA: left atrium, LAA: left atrial appendage.

## Computational modeling

CM is a method in which digital 3D reconstructions of any object can be illustrated in a 4D manner over time.[21] Used in biomedical engineering and sciences, CM fills the void that static models have in exemplifying the complex anatomic and physiologic interplay that occurs in real time. About 15 years ago, while in its infancy, computational models were created by simple manual drawings of geometric shapes. Today, the use of multi-modality imaging, such as CT and MRI in the case of cardiac models, is used for more refined and patient-specific modeling.[21] Through finite element analysis (FEA) and computational fluid dynamics (CFD), computational models can recreate stress and deformation of cardiac tissue, as well as to characterize the blood flow pattern in a patient's heart.[14,22]

The benefits of CM would be manifold, as it would allow for a way to take static cardiac images and bring them to life. This would give operators a greater understanding and sense of the physiologic environment in which they must operate. As such, CM may offer unique insights and even greater improvement in operator skill as well as procedural success.

## Artificial intelligence

AI is defined as the study of algorithms that give machines the ability to reason and perform functions such as problem-solving, object and word recognition, inference of world states, and decision-making.[23] AI has various applications across multiple disciplines, and it has recently found its way into improving precision-medicine and health care. Several procedural specialties have demonstrated the utility and accuracy offered by AI in training and procedure simulation, from general surgery, to anesthesiology, and even to neurosurgery, amongst many more.[23–25] Bissonnette and colleagues demonstrated the successful use of AI via machine learning algorithms in a surgical laminectomy simulation.[25] They showed that use of AI in their simulation achieved 97.6% accuracy in various metrics including the safety of the procedure, efficiency, motion of the tools, and coordination. Moreover, Engelhardt and colleagues used a deep neural network and recreation of the surgical scene to train operators for minimally invasive mitral valve repair, demonstrating its success in significantly improving their skills, understanding of complex mitral valve anatomy and surgical technique, and therefore, decreasing the time to crossing the learning curve.[26] As such, AI may have great potential in similarly improving accuracy, efficiency, and success in training for structural heart procedures.

## Benefits of Pre-Cath Laboratory Planning

### Patient selection

Many patients are not appropriate anatomical candidates for LAAO. Some individuals have a congenital absence of the LAA, others may have prior surgical and catheter interventions that preclude entry into the LAA, and lastly some patients may have an LAA thrombus present. Computed tomography is useful in pre-procedural planning to accurately characterize the above possible limitations or patient-specific contraindications to the procedure. Moreover, some patients may not be deemed a candidate for current generation LAAO devices due to LAA size and anatomy that is considered incompatible with their patient specific anatomy. However, in the setting of inadequate pre-procedural imaging, some patients may be deemed not a candidate for LAAO due to incomplete understanding of their patient specific anatomy, when in actuality they may have been anatomically suitable for LAAO by in-depth CT analysis.[27] Alternatively, some patients by pre-procedural 2D TEE or angiography may be deemed a candidate for LAAO, only to find intraprocedurally that the patient anatomy may not truly be amenable to any LAA occluder, rendering the patient with an aborted attempt at LAAO with failed attempt at stroke prevention.

*Thrombus visualization*

Cardiac CT is a noninvasive modality that offers important information not only of one's LAA anatomy but also of the presence or absence of LAA thrombus. Cardiac CT for LAAO is contrast-enhanced; therefore, a LAA thrombus is immediately visualized as a filling defect that should otherwise not be present. This mitigates the need for invasive tests such as TEE before LAAO for thrombus visualization and therefore mitigates health care spending and multiple medical encounters for the patient.

*Device sizing and procedure simulation*

It is clear that there exists an early-operator learning curve in LAAO device sizing and implantation.[14] Multi-modality imaging is extremely helpful in the appropriate sizing of the LAA, and accurate selection of the size of the LAAO device to be deployed. In fact, there is a significant difference in device size selection and less change in device size intraprocedurally with a greater success rate of device implantation in those with both CT and TEE guidance compared with TEE alone.[27] As shown in **Fig. 2**, there are various sizes offered for the WATCHMAN and WATCHMAN FLX devices. In cardiac CT, the LAA landing zone is appropriately sized at maximal LAA diastole or mid-late left ventricular systole (see **Fig. 2**). This is the moment in the cardiac cycle for which the LAA is at its largest, and therefore, an ideal phase for device sizing to mitigate risks of undersizing, and therefore, the risk of peridevice leaks and device embolization.[28]

Furthermore, CT images can be processed into 3D print models, which can offer finer detail and understanding of a patient's LAA anatomy. This can provide further granularity in sizing and successful mitigation of the above-mentioned risks. There is immense variability in LAA anatomy and structure from patient-to-patient, which is not readily seen in traditional echocardiographic techniques (see **Fig. 4**). This adds to further complexity in achieving success in LAAO, including device sizing, appropriate transseptal puncture, as well as device deployment.

CT imaging and 3D print models are extremely useful, particularly in LAAO procedure simulation. Printed models render a better understanding not only of complex LAA anatomy but also exhibit the visualization of left atrial size and dimensions for improved procedural planning. Accurate identification of the landing zone, simulation of transseptal puncture, appropriate catheter sizing for better deployment, and optimal C-arm angulations can all be determined with 3D print model-based simulation. In fact, one randomized study comparing LAAO guided by 3D-CT and 3D printing versus 2D TEE demonstrated significantly improved accuracy in device sizing (92% vs 27%, $P = .01$), improved procedural efficiency (55 $\pm$ 17 min vs 73 $\pm$ 24 min, $P < .05$), and fewer C-arm viewing projections (1.3 $\pm$ 1.2 vs 3.25 $\pm$ 2.52, $P = .05$).[15] Moreover, fewer devices and guide catheters were used in the former group compared with the 2D TEE cohort, namely due to preprocedural planning and simulation.[15]

As a result, early operator learning curves may significantly decrease with preprocedural 3D-CT and printed models.[7] Simulation offers the opportunity to teach trainees and early operators in a more effective way, further decreasing the time to crossing the learning curve. One study demonstrated a 100% success rate of LAAO with 1.245 devices per implantation attempt, compared with the average 1.8 devices per LAAO attempt (82% success rate) in the PROTECT-AF study.[7,29] Moreover, only 4 out of the 53 patients had peridevice leaks and no device embolization noted in the cohort.[7]

Although CT and 3D printing offer a more accurate understanding of the complexities of LAA anatomy, these offer static views without the live mechanics and physiology of a beating heart. Computational modeling opens a window into a more complete understanding of dynamic anatomy. Through computational simulation via methods such as FEA and CFD, these methods would provide further advantages in preprocedural planning. In addition to understanding static anatomy, computational modeling mimics reality with dynamic anatomy, offering a better understanding of real-time tissue deformation blood flow dynamics. Limitations to current widespread medical adaptation of computational modeling, such as FEA and CFD-based tools, include a paucity of easy-to-use medical grade softwares for medical teams in clinical practice, lack of clinical reimbursement, and absence of engineering expertise in integration of these tools to clinical practice.

Likewise, AI may even further individualize patient care when used in structural heart procedure planning. When used combination with 3D printing, AI may assist in the manufacturing of patient-specific anatomic replica, as well as real-time procedure simulation tailored to the patient's anatomy and physiology.[14] Through AI, patient-specific anatomy and physiology may be reconstructed to provide a framework for preprocedural planning and practice with instantaneous feedback in a much more realistic setting.

### Patient education

The use of 3D print models is effective not only in periprocedural planning but also may be considerably advantageous in patient education. Integration of 3D prints into clinical practice facilitates the shared decision-making between the patient and the physician. 3D print models can be used in the clinic setting to discuss therapeutic options in a much more visual, and therefore, effective way, rendering a much greater level of comprehension by the patient. This has led to further patient engagement in discussion with their physician, and therefore, better-informed decisions, and improved patient satisfaction. Application of 3D prints in clinical visits empowers patients with greater comprehension and knowledge of their disease, personal anatomy, and procedural recommendations for their care.[30–32]

### Limitations of Preprocedural Planning

Preprocedural planning is not critical to the successful development of an LAAO program in all hospitals. Operators and Interventional Imaging physician teams with significant preexisting expertise in LAAO procedures may not experience a significant additive value of periprocedural planning to their case outcomes. Additionally, depending on the size of the population served by the local health system, not all hospitals will have the same anticipated annual volume of LAAO procedures. Smaller sized LAAO programs may not have the financial reservoir necessary for the purchase of dedicated cardiac computed tomographic scanners for structural procedures. Additionally, in an era whereby reimbursement for cardiac coronary CT scanning is already challenging, reimbursement for the professional time necessary for performing intra or periprocedural structural heart CT planning is lacking. Modern intraprocedural techniques such as 3D angiography require training and experience, and both 3D angiography, as well as TEE fusion imaging, require capital equipment investments. Lastly, disparities in access to health care and reimbursement to new technologies vary by county and country delivering patient care and hence may limit Implanting Team's access to change their delivery of care.

### SUMMARY

Preprocedure planning for LAAO is critical to ensuring patient safety, procedural success, and optimal device outcomes for patient care. Pre-cath laboratory planning for LAAO can significantly improve procedural efficiency, accuracy, success, and therefore cost-effectiveness. In addition to multi-modality imaging, various modes of recreating cardiac anatomy and physiology, namely via 3D printing, computational modeling, and AI, can aid in significant improvements in achieving greater understanding of unique patient-specific anatomic and physiologic considerations in the procedural setting. The scalability of periprocedural planning in transcatheter interventions remains a discussion limited by regional practice patterns and solvent reimbursement strategies. As the LAAO procedure becomes more available globally, education on the importance of preprocedural LAAO planning is lagging. To ensure optimal safety and procedural success between the hands of experienced operators and new operators with new devices, preprocedural LAAO planning is invaluable.

### CLINICS CARE POINTS

- Current data support the use of pre-procedural CT as additive value for improving accuracy of LAA device sizing and procedural success.
- For any new LAAO implanter, incorporation of pre-procedural CT derived 3D printing and computational modeling decreases early operator learning curves associated with learning new devices and cardiac anatomies.
- Establishment of preprocedural imaging support protocols and pathways require institutional and societal investment in educational and reimbursment pathways for interventional imaging physicians to assist the Heart Team approach to LAAO procedures.

### DISCLOSURE

Dr D.D. Wang is a consultant for Edwards Lifesciences, Boston Scientific, Abbott, and Neochord. Dr D.D. Wang receives a research grant from Boston Scientific assigned to employer Henry Ford Health System not associated with this article. Dr T. De Potter consults for and received research grants not associated with this article from Boston Scientific, for which all invoices and payments are made directly to nonprofit "Cardiovascular Research Institute Aalst." All other authors report no relevant financial disclosures.

## REFERENCES

1. Sharma SP, Park P, Lakkireddy D. Left Atrial Appendages Occlusion: Current Status and Prospective. Korean Circ J 2018;48:692–704. Available at: http://www.ncbi.nlm.nih.gov/pubmed/30073807.

2. Blackshear JL, Odell JA. Appendage obliteration to reduce stroke in cardiac surgical patients with atrial fibrillation. Ann Thorac Surg 1996;61:755–9. Available at: http://www.ncbi.nlm.nih.gov/pubmed/8572814.

3. Reddy VY, Holmes D, Doshi SK, et al. Safety of percutaneous left atrial appendage closure: results from the Watchman Left Atrial Appendage System for Embolic Protection in Patients with AF (PROTECT AF) clinical trial and the Continued Access Registry. Circulation 2011;123:417–24. Available at: http://www.ncbi.nlm.nih.gov/pubmed/21242484.

4. Holmes DR, Kar S, Price MJ, et al. Prospective randomized evaluation of the Watchman Left Atrial Appendage Closure device in patients with atrial fibrillation versus long-term warfarin therapy: the PREVAIL trial. J Am Coll Cardiol 2014;64:1–12. Available at: http://www.ncbi.nlm.nih.gov/pubmed/24998121.

5. Boston Scientific. WATCHMAN Device Directions For Use. 2015. Available at: https://www.watchman.com/content/dam/watchman/downloads/dtr/watchman-matters-resources/WATCHMAN_Device_DFU_US.pdf.

6. Lockwood SM, Alison JF, Obeyesekere MN, et al. Imaging the left atrial appendage prior to, during, and after occlusion. JACC Cardiovasc Imaging 2011;4:303–6. Available at: http://www.ncbi.nlm.nih.gov/pubmed/21414580.

7. Wang DD, Eng M, Kupsky D, et al. Application of 3-Dimensional Computed Tomographic Image Guidance to WATCHMAN Implantation and Impact on Early Operator Learning Curve: Single-Center Experience. JACC Cardiovasc Interv 2016;9:2329–40. Available at: http://www.ncbi.nlm.nih.gov/pubmed/27884358.

8. Glikson M, Wolff R, Hindricks G, et al, ESC Scientific Document Group. EHRA/EAPCI expert consensus statement on catheter-based left atrial appendage occlusion - an update. EP Europace 2020;22(2):184. https://doi.org/10.1093/europace/euz258.

9. Spencer RJ, DeJong P, Fahmy P, et al. Changes in Left Atrial Appendage Dimensions Following Volume Loading During Percutaneous Left Atrial Appendage Closure. JACC Cardiovasc Interv 2015;8:1935–41. Available at: http://www.ncbi.nlm.nih.gov/pubmed/26738661.

10. Patel AR, Fatemi O, Norton PT, et al. Cardiac cycle-dependent left atrial dynamics: implications for catheter ablation of atrial fibrillation. Hear Rhythm 2008;5:787–93. Available at: http://www.ncbi.nlm.nih.gov/pubmed/18486563.

11. Shah PB, FGP Welt, Mahmud E, et al. Triage considerations for patients referred for structural heart disease intervention during the COVID-19 pandemic: An ACC/SCAI position statement. Catheter Cardiovasc Interv 2020;96:659–63. Available at: http://www.ncbi.nlm.nih.gov/pubmed/32251546.

12. Einstein AJ, Shaw LJ, Hirschfeld C, et al, INCAPS COVID Investigators Group. International Impact of COVID-19 on the Diagnosis of Heart Disease. J Am Coll Cardiol 2021;77:173–85. Available from: http://www.ncbi.nlm.nih.gov/pubmed/33446311.

13. Kaafarani M, Saw J, Daniels M, et al. Role of CT imaging in left atrial appendage occlusion for the WATCHMAN™ device. Cardiovasc Diagn Ther 2020;10:45–58.

14. Wang DD, Qian Z, Vukicevic M, et al. 3D printing, computational modeling, and artificial intelligence for structural heart disease. JACC Cardiovasc Imaging 2020;14(1):41–60. https://doi.org/10.1016/j.jcmg.2019.12.022.

15. Eng MH, Wang DD, Greenbaum AB, et al. Prospective, randomized comparison of 3-dimensional computed tomography guidance versus TEE data for left atrial appendage occlusion (PRO3DLAAO). Catheter Cardiovasc Interv 2018;92:401–7.

16. De Potter T, Chatzikyriakou S, Silva E, et al. A Pilot Study for Left Atrial Appendage Occlusion Guided by 3-Dimensional Rotational Angiography Alone. JACC Cardiovasc Interv 2018;11:223–4. Available at: http://www.ncbi.nlm.nih.gov/pubmed/29348017.

17. Balzer J, Zeus T, Hellhammer K, et al. Initial clinical experience using the EchoNavigator(®)-system during structural heart disease interventions. World J Cardiol 2015;7:562–70. Available at: http://www.ncbi.nlm.nih.gov/pubmed/26413233.

18. Ebelt H, Domagala T, Offhaus A, et al. Fusion Imaging of X-ray and Transesophageal Echocardiography Improves the Procedure of Left Atrial Appendage Closure. Cardiovasc Drugs Ther 2020;34:781–7. Available at: http://www.ncbi.nlm.nih.gov/pubmed/32761486.

19. Thaden JJ, Sanon S, Geske JB, et al. Echocardiographic and Fluoroscopic Fusion Imaging for Procedural Guidance: An Overview and Early Clinical Experience. J Am Soc Echocardiogr 2016;29:503–12. Available at: http://www.ncbi.nlm.nih.gov/pubmed/27021355.

20. Mo B-F, Wan Y, Alimu A, et al. Image fusion of integrating fluoroscopy into 3D computed tomography in guidance of left atrial appendage closure. Eur Hear Journal Cardiovasc Imaging 2021;22:92–101. Available at: http://www.ncbi.nlm.nih.gov/pubmed/31764982.

21. Lopez-Perez A, Sebastian R, Ferrero JM. Three-dimensional cardiac computational modelling: methods, features and applications. Biomed Eng 2015;14:35. Available at: http://www.ncbi.nlm.nih.gov/pubmed/25928297.

22. Aguado AM, Olivares AL, Yagüe C, et al. In silico Optimization of Left Atrial Appendage Occluder Implantation Using Interactive and Modeling Tools. Front Physiol 2019;10:237. Available at: http://www.ncbi.nlm.nih.gov/pubmed/30967786.

23. Hashimoto DA, Witkowski E, Gao L, et al. Artificial Intelligence in Anesthesiology: Current Techniques, Clinical Applications, and Limitations. Anesthesiology 2020;132:379–94. Available at: http://www.ncbi.nlm.nih.gov/pubmed/31939856.

24. Hashimoto DA, Rosman G, Rus D, et al. Artificial Intelligence in Surgery: Promises and Perils. Ann Surg 2018;268:70–6. Available at: http://www.ncbi.nlm.nih.gov/pubmed/29389679.

25. Bissonnette V, Mirchi N, Ledwos N, et al. Neurosurgical Simulation & Artificial Intelligence Learning Centre. Artificial Intelligence Distinguishes Surgical Training Levels in a Virtual Reality Spinal Task. J Bone Joint Surg Am 2019;101:e127. Available at: http://www.ncbi.nlm.nih.gov/pubmed/31800431.

26. Engelhardt S, Sauerzapf S, Brčić A, et al. Replicated mitral valve models from real patients offer training opportunities for minimally invasive mitral valve repair. Interact Cardiovasc Thorac Surg 2019;29:43–50. Available at: http://www.ncbi.nlm.nih.gov/pubmed/30783681.

27. So C-Y, Kang G, Villablanca PA, et al. Additive Value of Preprocedural Computed Tomography Planning Versus Stand-Alone Transesophageal Echocardiogram Guidance to Left Atrial Appendage Occlusion: Comparison of Real-World Practice. J Am Heart Assoc 2021;e020615. Available at: http://www.ncbi.nlm.nih.gov/pubmed/34398676.

28. Korsholm K, Berti S, Iriart X, et al. Expert Recommendations on Cardiac Computed Tomography for Planning Transcatheter Left Atrial Appendage Occlusion. JACC Cardiovasc Interv 2020;13:277–92.

29. Reddy VY, Sievert H, Halperin J, et al. PROTECT AF Steering Committee and Investigators. Percutaneous left atrial appendage closure vs warfarin for atrial fibrillation: a randomized clinical trial. JAMA 2014;312:1988–98. Available at: http://www.ncbi.nlm.nih.gov/pubmed/25399274.

30. Stewart JA, Wood L, Wiener J, et al. Visual teaching aids improve patient understanding and reduce anxiety prior to a colectomy. Am J Surg 2021;222(4):780–5. https://doi.org/10.1016/j.amjsurg.2021.01.029.

31. Kliot T, Zygourakis CC, Imershein S, et al. The impact of a patient education bundle on neurosurgery patient satisfaction. Surg Neurol Int 2015;6:S567–72. Available at: http://www.ncbi.nlm.nih.gov/pubmed/26664909.

32. Oudkerk Pool MD, Hooglugt J-LQ, Schijven MP, et al. Review of Digitalized Patient Education in Cardiology: A Future Ahead? Cardiology 2021;1–9. Available at: http://www.ncbi.nlm.nih.gov/pubmed/33550295.

# The Case for Intracardiac Echo to Guide Left Atrial Appendage Closure

Mohamad Alkhouli, MD[a],*,
Jens Erik Nielsen-Kudsk, MD, DMSc[b]

## KEYWORDS

- Atrial fibrillation • Stroke prevention • Left atrial appendage closure • Intracardiac echo
- Transesophageal echo

## KEY POINTS

- TEE is currently the predominant imaging method to guide LAAC.
- ICE has emerged an a safe, and cost-effective alternative to TEE in guiding LAAC.
- Several issues need to be considered when starting an ICE-guided LAAC program including the use of pre-procedural CTA, the commitment and routine use of ICE, and the use of a simplified imaging protocol.

Stroke prevention is the cornerstone of nonvalvular atrial fibrillation management.[1] Oral anticoagulation (OAC) is the standard stroke prevention strategy in most patients. However, many patients are not on effective OAC because of perceived or experienced side effects, prohibitive cost, and noncompliance.[2] Left atrial appendage closure (LAAC) has emerged as a promising strategy to address this unmet need. With the growing acceptance and utilization of LAAC worldwide, efforts have been made to streamline the procedure and enhance its safety and efficacy. As part of these efforts, minimally invasive methods to perform LAAC without general anesthesia or under light to moderate sedation and with intracardiac echocardiography (ICE)[3] guidance have been developed.[4] Yet, wide adoption of ICE-guided LAAC remains hindered by the concerns about the learning curve, the incremental cost, the limitations of the current ICE technology, and the lack of imaging standards. Most LAAC procedures continue to be performed under general anesthesia with transesophageal echocardiography (TEE) guidance. In this article, we review the issues related to the routine use of ICE in LAAC and provide a concise guide for new users interested in the adoption of ICE in their LAAC practice.

## RATIONAL FOR ICE-GUIDED LAAC

Despite the increasing interest in ICE to guide structural heart disease (SHD) interventions, a common question arises when this topic is debated: TEE is excellent, why ICE? There is little debate that TEE is an excellent platform for guiding LAAC and other SHD procedures. Indeed, TEE enjoys several advantages: (a) TEE was the imaging modality used in randomized trials for preprocedural planning, procedural guidance, and postprocedural surveys; (b) TEE allows multiplanar and 3D imaging, which can be essential for a comprehensive assessment of the highly variable left atrial appendage (LAA) anatomies; (c) TEE is inexpensive, and there is a widespread experience with it worldwide; (d) TEE guidance allows the operator to focus on the interventional aspect of the procedure and

---

Funding: none.
[a] Department of Cardiology, Mayo Clinic School of Medicine, 200 First Street Southwest, Rochester, MN 55905, USA; [b] Department of Cardiology, Aarhus University Hospital, Palle Juul-Jensens Boulevard 99, DK-8200 Aarhus N, Denmark
* Corresponding author.
*E-mail address:* Alkhouli.Mohamad@mayo.edu

2211-7458/22/© 2021 Elsevier Inc. All rights reserved.

not be potentially distracted by the imaging component; and (e) the instruction for use of the Food and Drug Administration approved LAAC devices to date (Watchman & Watchman FLX; Boston Scientific, Marlborough, MA) require TEE imaging in 4 different views to ensure acceptable position, anchor, seal, and compression (P.A.S.S criteria).

On the other hand, ICE has major advantages that make it an excellent alternative for TEE:

*First*, patients referred for LAAC are elderly, have a high burden of comorbidities, and a high prevalence of frailty.[3] Hence, avoidance of general anesthesia in these patients would plausibly yield several benefits. Although this has not been specifically studied in the LAAC population, data from comparable SHD populations support this notion. Indeed, moderate sedation among patients undergoing transcatheter aortic valve replacement has been shown to be associated with lower mortality, shorter hospital stays, and more frequent discharge to home compared with procedures performed with general anesthesia.[5] Considering the inability to guide LAAC with surface echocardiography, ICE is uniquely positioned to provide an alternative to TEE that precludes the use of general anesthesia in this vulnerable population. Proponents of TEE suggest that pediatric (and even) adult-size probes can be used to guide LAAC under moderate sedation.[6,7] However, many institutions have policies that mandate general anesthesia for prolonged TEE imaging in supine patients regardless of the TEE technology used. Furthermore, pediatric probes lack X-plane and 3D capabilities, which would deprive TEE from some of its major advantages over ICE and they offer lower imaging resolution than adult probes.

*Second*, TEE is not without risk, especially in predominantly elderly and frail populations. Reported TEE-related complications with interventional procedures in the catheterization laboratory are more frequent compared with what was previously reported in the operating room or in the ambulatory settings.[8,9] A recent study that compared upper gastrointestinal endoscopy performed before and immediately after TEE-guided SHD interventions in 50 patients found a new injury in 86% of patients (43/50) with complex lesions in 40% (20/50) of these patients.[8] The risk of complex injury increased for each 10 minutes increment in imaging time (odds ratio [OR] 1.27: 95% confidence interval [CI] 1.01 to 1.59), and poor imaging quality (OR 4.93; 95% CI 1.10–22.02).

*Third*, ICE can be used in patients with gastroesophageal and hepatic disorders in whom TEE is often contraindicated. A typical example is patients with hepatic cirrhosis and esophageal varices who are often referred for LAAC because of intolerance to OAC.

*Fourth*, ICE provides excellent imaging of the interatrial septum facilitating optimal transseptal puncture. It is often superior to TEE, especially for imaging the inferoposterior part of the septum, which is the preferred site of puncture for most LAAC cases.

*Fifth*, ICE facilitates a much-improved workflow in the catheterization laboratory. Rather than scheduling at least 3 operators (interventionalist, anesthesiologist, and echocardiographer) for a single case, the case could be performed with a single operator. An assistant to the primary operator (eg, trainee, technician, etc) is usually present regardless of the utilized imaging modality. Early comparative data of ICE versus TEE have shown significantly shorter room time with ICE-guided procedures.[10–12]

*Sixth*, TEE often yields suboptimal imaging because of the wide variability in the size, shape, and orientation of the LAA. Although ICE may be suggested as a substitute to TEE in selected challenging scenarios, nonroutine use of ICE is problematic as it limits the experience with ICE imaging, which severely hinders the ability to tackle challenging-only cases. Furthermore, the interest in and the use of ICE continues to grow in other SHD procedures where TEE routinely underperforms (eg, tricuspid valve edge-to-edge repair).[13] The increasing experience associated with adopting ICE for LAAC will likely have a positive impact on other SHD interventions.[4]

With these potential advantages in mind, a prospective adaptor of ICE would still want to know if there are data to support that ICE-guided LAAC is safe, effective, and at least cost-neutral.

## DATA SUPPORTING ICE-GUIDED LAAC

Published reports of ICE-guided LAAC can be traced back to 2007.[14,15] However, these were reports of a small number of cases that used both TEE and ICE for procedural guidance with the ICE probe positioned in the coronary sinus. The first LAAC guided with ICE as a standalone imaging modality was published by MacDonald and colleagues in 2010.[16] In this case, ICE was positioned in the pulmonary artery inside a Mullins sheath (Medtronic, Minneapolis, MN) and successfully guided the procedure. Later, more accounts of ICE-guided LAAC from the right side of the heart emerged. In 2014, Berti and colleagues reported a dual center experience of

LAAC guided solely by ICE positioned in the right atrium or the coronary sinus.[17] In this report, technical success was achieved in 117 of 121 patients (96.7%) with a major complication rate of 3.3%. Unfortunately, right-sided ICE imaging for LAAC lacked reproducibility in subsequent studies. Therefore, the focus has quickly shifted to assessing the feasibility of LAAC guided with an ICE probe in the left atrium (LA).

In 2016, Frangieh illustrated a 100% technical success rate of a series of 32 patients who underwent LAAC guided with the ICE probe advanced to the LA through a single transseptal puncture.[18] In 2017, Korsholm and colleagues compared the outcomes of TEE versus ICE-guided LAAC in 216 patients at a referral Danish center.[12] Compared with TEE-guided procedures, ICE-guided LAAC procedures were associated with a similar success rate (99.1%), but less contrast use and shorter procedural time. Complication rates, peridevice leak, and the prevalence of residual atrial septal defects were comparable between the 2 groups. Later, data from 2 European registries (multicenter Italian registry and the Amulet observational study) similarly showed comparable success and complication rates with TEE versus ICE-guided LAAC, although procedural times were slightly shorter in the TEE arm likely due to the learning curve of ICE imaging at new adapting centers.[19,20]

Data on ICE use in LAAC procedures in the United States remain limited. Hemam and colleagues compared TEE versus ICE-guided LAAC in 104 patients at 3 US electrophysiology laboratories.[11] In this study, ICE was used selectively in a limited number of patients at the operators' discretion, and most LAAC remained guided by TEE. Similar to the previously published European experiences, ICE guidance was associated with high success rate and improved procedural turnaround time with no difference in success rate or adverse events. Total hospital charges were similar in both groups. Alkhouli and colleagues compared clinical, efficiency metrics, and cost data before and after switching from TEE-guided LAAC to routine ICE-guided LAAC in all comers.[10] No exclusion criteria for ICE guidance based on LAA anatomy or clinical comorbidities were applied at the time of transition. Procedural success and complication rates were similar. Hospital charges were higher in the ICE cohort, but professional fees were higher in the TEE cohort, yielding a similar overall cost in both groups.

More recently, additional reports emerged confirming the safety and efficacy of ICE guidance for LAAC using second generation occluder devices (Watchman FLX, Boston Scientific).[21,22] In aggregate, there are ample data supporting the feasibility, safety, and efficacy of ICE-guided LAAC. Furthermore, 2 prospective studies (I Can sEe Left Atrial Appendage [ICELAA] Clinical Study [NCT04196335], and the ICE WATCHMAN study [NCT04569734]) are underway aiming to provide a standardized imaging technique and validation of ICE device release criteria (ICE P.A.S.S).

## TIPS FOR SUCCESSFUL ICE-GUIDED LAAC PROGRAM

Venues to learn ICE-guided LAAC have been limited because of industry hesitation to embrace ICE until more safety data are collected. Nonetheless, the interest in ICE is rapidly growing considering (1) the accumulation of safety and efficacy data on ICE-guided LAAC; (2) the Food and Drug Administration approval of potentially groundbreaking 4D ICE technologies (VeriSight; Philips, Andover, MA and NuVision; Biosense Webster, Irvine, CA); and (3) The increasing interest in avoiding aerosolized procedures brought by the COVID-19 pandemic.[23] Hence, we anticipate that more structured ICE learning opportunities will become available for interested operators both at major conferences and as standalone workshops. In addition to subscribing to such educational occasions, we offer the following tips on factors that we found essential for starting and growing a successful ICE-guided LAAC program:

1. Adoption of cardiac computed tomography (CCT). The superiority of CCT assessment of LAA anatomy has been demonstrated in multiple studies.[24] In addition, new dedicated software (eg, TruPlan, Boston Scientific, 3mensio) allow not only LAA measurement but also the prediction of optimal transseptal access location, sheath selection, and ICE simulation. Consensus recommendations on the ideal methods for imaging acquisition and interpretation have been published.[25] In our practice, CCT is the imaging modality of choice pre-LAAO in patients without advanced renal insufficiency.
2. Commitment. Like any new technique, integrating ICE in SHD interventional practice requires the operator's commitment. The major 2 components of the learning curve are crossing the intra-atrial septum with the ICE catheter and navigating it in the LA. The learning curve to master these steps in our experience

ranges between 10 and 20 cases. Electrophysiologists are facile with these techniques and partnering with them might offer an excellent opportunity to flatten this learning curve. Operators might also benefit from adopting ICE as a useful tool for a variety of SHD procedures rather than learning ICE guidance for a specific procedure (eg, LAAC).[26] Experience gained with ICE to guide PFO and ASD closures is highly valuable in the learning process of ICE-guided LAAC.

3. Use ICE routinely. Although reverting to TEE guidance could be justified in some cases (eg, combined valve and LAAC procedure, closure of persistent leak after LAAC), selective use of ICE in a limited number of patients yields suboptimal outcomes. In our practice, we use ICE in all patients who have suitable anatomy for closure regardless of the size and shape of the LAA. We suggest starting with simple LAA anatomies at first with proctoring if feasible, but gradually adopting an all-comer strategy to optimize clinical outcomes and realize the full benefits of ICE-guided LAAC.

4. Use a simplified but a systematic approach. A minimum of 2 views are needed to ensure a detailed survey of the device.[10] A 3-view approach from the LA was recommended in a recent expert consensus, especially for new ICE users: (1) left upper pulmonary vein

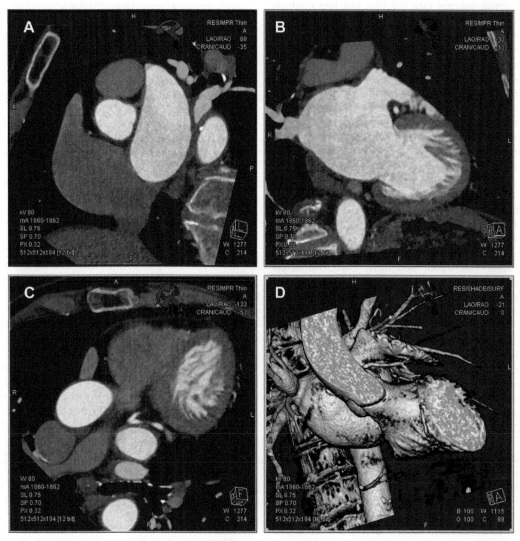

Fig. 1. Preprocedural assessment with cardiac computed tomography. (A-C) Orthogonal views and multiplanar reconstruction of the left atrial appendage. (D) 3D view of the left atrial appendage.

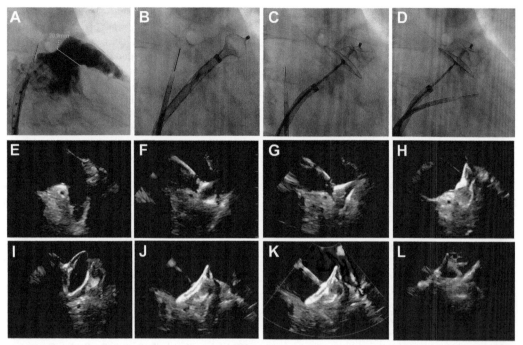

**Fig. 2.** Step-by-step ICE-guided LAAC with an Amulet device. Top panel: (*A*) Angiography showing a chicken wing LAA anatomy. (*B–D*) Illustration of the ICE positions in the 3 standard views: (*B*) left upper pulmonary vein (LUPV) view, (*C*) mid-LA view, and (*D*) supra-mitral view. Middle panel: (*E–H*) LAA from the LUPV; Amulet lobe in the ball configuration; lobe in the triangular configuration and lobe deployed in the neck of the LAA. Lower panel: (*I–L*) Amulet disc being deployed (American football configuration); disc fully deployed; color Doppler without signs of peridevice leakage; the Amulet device seen in the supramitral view.

view, (2) mid-LA view, and (3) supramitral view (**Figs. 1** and **2**).[20]

5. Consider ICE is a distinct imaging modality. A common observation with new ICE adaptors is the tendency to seek a direct head-to-head comparison with TEE. We believe that this strategy is counterproductive. There is a limited number of studies that compare and validate TEE and ICE imaging in the same patients. In addition, imaging with ICE as a stand-alone modality has been shown to be safe and effective in guiding LAAO regardless of its comparability to TEE. Furthermore, studies designed to validate the use of dedicated ICE P.A.S.S criteria for device release are underway (ICELAA and ICE WATCHMAN) and would hopefully increase operators' comfort with ICE-guided LAAO.

## SUMMARY

Patients who are good candidates for LAAC are often poor candidates for general anesthesia because of age, multimorbidity, and frailty. ICE makes it possible to do LAAC in local anesthesia. It is a safe and effective imaging alternative to TEE for guiding LAAC. ICE-guided LAAC is associated with shorter procedure time, improved workflow, and possibly clinical benefits. Newer ICE technology will further shorten the learning curve and allow new operators to seemingly adopt a predominately ICE-guided LAAC strategy.

## CLINICS CARE POINTS

- ICE provides an effective method to guide LAAC in contemporary practice.
- Current data show that ICE-guided LAAC is a safe and cost-effective strategy when compared with TEE-guided LAAC.
- Advantages of ICE-guided LAAC include the elimination of risks associated with general anesthesia and TEE, and the fascillation of a shorter hospital stay.

## DISCLOSURE

Dr M. Alkhouli served on the advisory board for Boston Scientific, Philips, Abbott, and Biosense Webster. Dr

J.E. Nielsen-Kudsk is a consultant and proctor for Abbott and Boston Scientific.

## REFERENCES

1. Alkhouli M, Noseworthy PA, Rihal CS, et al. Stroke prevention in nonvalvular atrial fibrillation: a stakeholder perspective. J Am Coll Cardiol 2018;71:2790–801.

2. Holmes DR Jr, Alkhouli M, Reddy V. Left atrial appendage occlusion for the unmet clinical needs of stroke prevention in nonvalvular atrial fibrillation. Mayo Clin Proc 2019;94:864–74.

3. Freeman JV, Varosy P, Price MJ, et al. The NCDR left atrial appendage occlusion registry. J Am Coll Cardiol 2020;75:1503–18.

4. Alkhouli M, Hijazi ZM, Holmes DR Jr, et al. Intracardiac echocardiography in structural heart disease interventions. JACC Cardiovasc Interv 2018;11:2133–47.

5. Butala NM, Chung M, Secemsky EA, et al. Conscious sedation versus general anesthesia for transcatheter aortic valve replacement: variation in practice and outcomes. JACC Cardiovasc Interv 2020;13:1277–87.

6. Piayda K, Hellhammer K, Nielsen-Kudsk JE, et al. Clinical outcomes of patients undergoing percutaneous left atrial appendage occlusion in general anaesthesia or conscious sedation: data from the prospective global Amplatzer Amulet Occluder Observational Study. BMJ Open 2021;11:e040455.

7. Maarse M, Wintgens LIS, Klaver MN, et al. Transoesophageal echocardiography guidance with paediatric probes in adults undergoing left atrial appendage occlusion. EuroIntervention 2021;17:93–6.

8. Freitas-Ferraz AB, Bernier M, Vaillancourt R, et al. Safety of Transesophageal Echocardiography to Guide Structural Cardiac Interventions. J Am Coll Cardiol 2020;75:3164–73.

9. Freitas-Ferraz AB, Rodes-Cabau J, Junquera Vega L, et al. Transesophageal echocardiography complications associated with interventional cardiology procedures. Am Heart J 2020;221:19–28.

10. Alkhouli M, Chaker Z, Alqahtani F, et al. Outcomes of routine intracardiac echocardiography to guide left atrial appendage occlusion. JACC Clin Electrophysiol 2020;6:393–400.

11. Hemam ME, Kuroki K, Schurmann PA, et al. Left atrial appendage closure with the Watchman device using intracardiac vs transesophageal echocardiography: Procedural and cost considerations. Heart Rhythm 2019;16:334–42.

12. Korsholm K, Jensen JM, Nielsen-Kudsk JE. Intracardiac echocardiography from the left atrium for procedural guidance of transcatheter left atrial appendage occlusion. JACC Cardiovasc Interv 2017;10:2198–206.

13. Alkhouli M, Eleid MF, Michellena H, et al. Complementary roles of intracardiac and transoesophageal echocardiography in transcatheter tricuspid interventions. EuroIntervention 2020;15:1514–5.

14. Ho IC, Neuzil P, Mraz T, et al. Use of intracardiac echocardiography to guide implantation of a left atrial appendage occlusion device (PLAATO). Heart Rhythm 2007;4:567–71.

15. Mraz T, Neuzil P, Mandysova E, et al. Role of echocardiography in percutaneous occlusion of the left atrial appendage. Echocardiography 2007;24:401–4.

16. MacDonald ST, Newton JD, Ormerod OJ. Intracardiac echocardiography off piste? Closure of the left atrial appendage using ICE and local anesthesia. Catheter Cardiovasc Interv 2011;77:124–7.

17. Berti S, Paradossi U, Meucci F, et al. Periprocedural intracardiac echocardiography for left atrial appendage closure: a dual-center experience. JACC Cardiovasc Interv 2014;7:1036–44.

18. Frangieh AH, Alibegovic J, Templin C, et al. Intracardiac versus transesophageal echocardiography for left atrial appendage occlusion with watchman. Catheter Cardiovasc Interv 2017;90:331–8.

19. Nielsen-Kudsk JE, Berti S, De Backer O, et al. Use of intracardiac compared with transesophageal echocardiography for left atrial appendage occlusion in the amulet observational study. JACC Cardiovasc Interv 2019;12:1030–9.

20. Berti S, Pastormerlo LE, Santoro G, et al. Intracardiac versus transesophageal echocardiographic guidance for left atrial appendage occlusion: the LAAO Italian Multicenter Registry. JACC Cardiovasc Interv 2018;11:1086–92.

21. Turagam MK, Neuzil P, Petru J, et al. Intracardiac echocardiography-guided implantation of the Watchman FLX left atrial appendage closure device. J Cardiovasc Electrophysiol 2021;32:717–25.

22. Korsholm K, Samaras A, Andersen A, et al. The Watchman FLX Device: First European Experience and Feasibility of Intracardiac Echocardiography to Guide Implantation. JACC Clin Electrophysiol 2020;6:1633–42.

23. Alkhouli M, Coylewright M, Holmes DR. Will the COVID-19 epidemic reshape cardiology? Eur Heart J Qual Care Clin Outcomes 2020;6(3):217–20.

24. Korsholm K, Jensen JM, Nielsen-Kudsk JE. Cardiac computed tomography for left atrial appendage occlusion: acquisition, analysis, advantages, and limitations. Interv Cardiol Clin 2018;7:229–42.

25. Korsholm K, Berti S, Iriart X, et al. Expert recommendations on cardiac computed tomography for planning transcatheter left atrial appendage occlusion. JACC Cardiovasc Interv 2020;13:277–92.

26. Raphael CE, Alkhouli M, Maor E, et al. Building blocks of structural intervention: a novel modular paradigm for procedural training. Circ Cardiovasc Interv 2017;10:e005686.

# Follow Up imaging After Left Atrial Appendage Occlusion–Something or Nothing and for How Long?

Thomas Nestelberger, MD[a,b,c], Mesfer Alfadhel, MD[a],
Cameron McAlister, MD[a], Jacqueline Saw, MD[a,d,e,*]

**KEYWORDS**

- Left atrial appendage closure • Follow-up • Imaging
- Cardiac computer tomography angiography • Transesophageal echocardiography

**KEY POINTS**

- Peri-device leaks, device-related thrombus, and device embolization are rare but potential harmful complications after left atrial appendage closure procedures.
- Routine postprocedural imaging with transesophageal echocardiography is the most commonly used imaging modality for follow-up surveillance performed 1 to 6 months after the procedure.
- Cardiac computed tomography angiography offers a high-resolution 3-dimensional imaging with a reproducibility and low interoperator variability and may a viable alternative to transesophageal echocardiography for postimplant device surveillance of left atrial appendage occlusion.

## INTRODUCTION

Atrial fibrillation (AF) is the most common cardiac arrhythmia with current prevalence estimated at 1.5% to 2% of the general population and affecting ~9% of adults older than 80 years.[1] Notably, the presence of nonvalvular AF is associated with a 4- to 5-fold increased risk of ischemic stroke.[2] Over the last 2 decades alternative methods for prevention of thromboembolic events have been emerged, with the most important alternative being left atrial appendage (LAA) occlusion (LAAO). The LAA is the major source of nonvalvular AF-related thromboembolism, as more than 90% of these clots reside in the LAA.[3] Technological innovation has led to the development of transcatheter-based, minimally invasive devices for LAAO. The outcomes of patients after successful implantation of LAAO device can be affected by device position, presence of peri-device leak (PDL) and device-related thrombus (DRT). Therefore, routine surveillance imaging is necessary.[4]

The use of multimodality pre-peri and postprocedural imaging including cardiac computer tomography angiography (CCTA), transesophageal echocardiography (TEE), or intracardiac echocardiography (ICE) in conjunction with fluoroscopy is critical for procedural safety and implant success. A transthoracic echocardiogram should be performed before discharge to ensure that the device has remained in

Funding: This review was not funded.
[a] Division of Cardiology, Vancouver General Hospital, University of British Columbia, 2775 Laurel Street, Level 9, Vancouver, BC V5Z1M9, Canada; [b] Cardiovascular Research Institute Basel (CRIB), University Hospital Basel, University of Basel, Basel, Switzerland; [c] Department of Cardiology, University Hospital Basel, University of Basel, Basel, Switzerland; [d] Vancouver General Hospital, Basel, British Columbia, Canada; [e] University of British Columbia, 2775 Laurel Street, 9th Floor, Vancouver, British Columbia V5Z 1M9, Canada
* Corresponding author.
*E-mail address:* jsaw@mail.ubc.ca

2211-7458/22/© 2021 Elsevier Inc. All rights reserved.

| Abbreviations | |
|---|---|
| PDL | Peri-device Leak |
| DRT | Device Related Thrombus |

position in the LAA and to exclude pericardial effusion.[4] After discharge, device surveillance is recommended 6 to 12 weeks post-LAAO with either TEE or CCTA, primarily to assess for DRT and PDL (residual LAA patency).[4] If the patient is at risk for developing DRT (eg, noncompliance with antithrombotic therapy post-LAAO, deep implant, poor left ventricular function), then repeat device surveillance imaging at 6 to 12 months is also recommended.[5] Regardless of the device type, all studies report DRT formation and incomplete LAA coverage as the most common complications during follow-up after LAAO. Although TEE is the most used technique for follow-up in most centers, the high spatial resolution and noninvasive multiplanar capability of contemporary contrast-enhanced electrocardiography-gated multidetector CCTA has led this modality to be increasingly used in many institutions for assessing procedural success and complications post-LAAO.

### Left Atrial Appendage Anatomy

The LAA usually arises as a fingerlike projection from the left atrium and forms part of the left border of the heart, superior to the left ventricle and inferior to the main pulmonary trunk.[6] The tip or apex of the LAA can vary in position but usually points anteriorly and superiorly coming into close apposition with the proximal left anterior descending coronary artery, the proximal circumflex artery, and the pulmonary trunk.[7] It may point inferiorly and posteriorly or behind the aorta into the transverse pericardial sinus. Several different shapes have been described, but for device deployment purposes, the LAA can be considered as multilobed with an obvious bend (chicken wing morphology), single lobed without a bend (windsock morphology), multilobed without an obvious bend or dominant lobe (cauliflower shape), or multilobed without an obvious bend but with a dominant lobe (cactus shape).[8] Different morphologies may be associated with different risks of thromboembolism, with the chicken wing morphology thought to confer the lowest risk.[9] The various shapes and sizes of LAA and orientation of the atrial ostium may contribute to incomplete LAA closure.[10]

### Imaging Acquisition with Transesophageal Echocardiography and Computer Tomography Angiography

TEE is regarded as the gold standard for device surveillance following LAAO, especially for the diagnosis of DRT.[4] However, CCTA is an appealing alternative because of its noninvasive nature. Despite TEE having higher temporal resolution, cardiac CT has superior spatial resolution, is isotropic by nature with 3-dimensional and multiplanar capabilities and is less operator dependent. The aim of TEE or CCTA during follow-up after LAAO is to assess device position, PDL and DRT. For TEE imaging acquisition, sedation is necessary in most of the patients, and exclusion of absolute and relative contraindications such as esophageal strictures and varices is important to ensure safe and high-quality examinations.[11] DRT by TEE is usually described as a homogenous echodense mass visible in multiple planes with independent motion and adherence to the atrial surface of the LAAO device, whereas PDL is described as the width of the color Doppler jet with a Nyquist scale set between 20 and 50 cm/s from the left atrium to the LAA. Definition of PDL using TEE varied across several studies and registries.[10,12–16]

Imaging acquisition with CCTA is commonly performed as a prospective electrocardiogram-gated scan using a high-pitch single-heartbeat spiral acquisition protocol (Table 1). For LAA assessment, systolic phase at 30% to 40% of RR interval is imaged for largest dimensions. Tube voltage is set between 70 and 150 kV depending on body weight. Automated tube current modulation should be used. Based on a test bolus, a single contrast injection (350 mg I/mL iodine concentration) should be administered through an antecubital vein at flow rates of 5 to 6 mL/s, followed by a 50 mL saline flush. The scan should be performed with patients in a euvolemic state, with oral hydration or intravenous saline given before scanning, as both the size and volume of the LAA change with volume status.[17] Images are reconstructed with a 0.5 to 0.75 mm slice thickness.[18] The processed images can be assessed for atrial-side device thrombus, residual contrast leak (patency) into the LAA, device embolization, device positioning, pericardial effusion, the presence of peri-device gap,

**Table 1**
Suggested cardiac computer tomography angiography protocol for left atrial appendage closure procedures with Toshiba or Siemens scanners

| | |
|---|---|
| Gating | Prospective ECG-gated |
| Tube potential | 100 kV for BMI <30,120 kV if BMI >30 |
| Tube current | 300–500 mA with ECG tube current modulation |
| Scan direction | Cranial to caudal |
| Scan volume | Heart to diaphragm (14–16 cm) |
| Size | Images reconstructed to 0.5 and 0.6 mm with 40% overlap, 512 × 512 mm matrix, reconstruction field of view 250 mm |
| Detector collimation | 320 × 0.5 mm Toshiba or 128 × 0.6 mm Siemens |
| Cardiac phase reconstruction | Relative triggering 30%–40% of RR interval or absolute triggering 250 ms after R wave |
| Contrast bolus tracking | Sure Start (Toshiba), Cardiac Definition (Siemens), or CareDose (Siemens Somatom) |
| IV contrast injection | 50–80 cc Optiray contrast, followed by 50 cc 30% contrast/70% saline mixture, and final 30 cc saline chaser |
| Flow rate | 5–6 mL/s |
| Heart rate | No restrictions |
| β-blocker and nitrates | Not required |

*Abbreviations:* BMI, body mass index; ECG, electrocardiogram; IV, intravenous.

and device lobe dimensions. Lobe compression (%) can be calculated as: [(manufacturer device diameter 2 measured diameter)/manufacturer device diameter] × 100%. Residual leak (patency) into the LAA is assessed by measurements of the linear attenuation coefficient (Hounsfield unit, HU) in the LAA distal to the device and comparison of contrast density to surrounding cardiac chambers.[19]

For the assessment of LAA thrombus in the absence of an LAAO device, the sensitivity of CCTA was reported between 29% and 100%, with specificity 67% to 100% and positive predictive value 12% to 100%.[20] A recent meta-analysis of 19 studies showed a mean sensitivity of 96% and specificity of 92%.[21] However, the most consistent finding was a high negative predictive value ranging between 96% and 100% across studies.[21] As a consequence, most investigators conclude that patients without filling defects on cardiac CT do not require additional TEE examination.[22] There are limited data on the use of CCTA to detect DRT post-LAAO, although 2 large case series had reported that all DRT found on TEE were also observed on CCTA, with some reassurance that CCTA is likely adequate to assess DRT.[18,23]

Although CCTA seems to be a valuable alternative to TEE, the limitations of cardiac CT imaging should be acknowledged. Contrast administration may be problematic in some patients, reducing the generalized feasibility of cardiac CT. In addition, radiation exposure might be a concern. Previous studies have reported mean radiation exposure between 3.5 and 6.6 mSv.[19,20] The risk of contrast-induced nephropathy is another limitation. In most studies the reported incidence of contrast-induced acute kidney injury was less than 1% in standard patients undergoing elective contrast-enhanced imaging and less than 4% in patients with chronic kidney disease.[24]

**Peri-Device Leak After Percutaneous Device Closure**

The shape and size of the LAA is variable, and the orifice is typically elliptical (68.9%), whereas percutaneous LAAO devices are circular by design.[24] This mismatch in geometry provides the potential for incomplete LAA occlusion and residual PDL.[15] In addition, the orientation of the LAA ostium and the proximal surface of the device may also be malaligned during deployment with resultant PDL. The definition of severity of PDL is arbitrary depending on the devices and imaging modalities. This lack of standardized criteria for leaks may lead to controversies regarding its relation to thromboembolic events.[10] A PDL is defined as the presence of flow past the edge of an implanted device into the LAA, as determined by color Doppler on TEE or the presence of contrast within the LAA on CCTA.[13,25] The definition of significant leak ranges from a 1 to 5 mm width of residual flow (leak) on color Doppler using TEE. For the Watchman device, a greater than 5-mm PDL at 45-day TEE was considered significant and may warrant continuation of oral anticoagulation. For the Amplatzer Cardiac Plug or Amplatzer Amulet devices, PDL is considered as the presence of a color jet around the device lobe on multiplane images of TEE.[13] Other studies suggested a leak around the disk and lobe on CCTA.[26] The incidence of PDL has been reported in a range of 5% to 32% at a 1-year follow-up, depending on its definition and different devices.[12,13,15,25,27] The predictors of PDL after LAAO are not clearly identified, although there are reports showing that device compression rate of less than 10% was associated with PDL.[25] The correlation of PDL or residual flow to clinical events is not well established. In the PROTECT-AF trial with the Watchman device, PDL was present in 40.9%, 33.8%, and 32.1% of the patients at 45 days, 6 months, and 12 months after Watchman device implantation, respectively.[12] In this study, residual PDL was not associated with an increased risk of thromboembolism regardless of the size of the leak (<1, 1–3, and >3 mm). However, the investigators emphasized that the confidence of the results was limited due to small sample size or low event rates in the study. In addition, in PDL greater than 3 mm, oral anticoagulation was continued, whereas antiplatelet therapy alone was prescribed in smaller leaks, which might have influenced the thrombus rate in these cases. Furthermore, the clinical implication of larger PDLs (>5 mm width) was not evaluated in this study. More recently the novel Watchman FLX device was evaluated in a single-arm Food and Drug Administration approval study in 400 patients, which reported only 17.2% and 10.5% of patients had any peri-device flow less than or equal to 5 mm in diameter at 45-day and 12-month follow-up, and no patient had a jet size greater than 5 mm. Accordingly, ~90% had no detectable PDL.[28]

PDL in patients who received the Amplatzer Amulet device was assessed in a prospective multicenter study.[29] At 12 months after device implantation, PDL was noted in 11.6% to 12.5% of patients on follow-up TEE, which was lower than PDL incidence of the Watchman device (32.1%).[13,29] The "lobe-and-disc" design of the Amplatzer Amulet device may cover the orifice of the LAA and may result in lower incidence of PDL compared with the "single-lobe" design of the Watchman device. Severe PDL (>5 mm or multiple jets) was observed in 0.6% of the overall cohort (2/339) and in 5% of all reported PDLs (2/39). However, no independent predictors of PDL or clinical outcomes were identified in this study due to the low study power. In an imaging study by Nguyen and colleagues[25] CCTA detected 56.7% (17/30) of PDL from mixed devices (Watchman, Amplatzer Cardiac Plug, and Amulet). In this study, the incidence of major adverse cardiac event was quantitatively higher in patients with PDL, but the difference was not statistically significant between patients with PDL versus without PDL (12 vs 4.3%, P = .3), but the sample size was small. Although it is not considered a PDL, persistent large accessory lobes adjacent to an LAA that remain unclosed by the occluding device can cause thromboembolism. This event is more common for devices that use the "plug principle," such as Watchman occluders. Devices that use the "pacifier principle," meaning they include a proximal disc, can cover this accessory lobe and, therefore, may have a decreased incidence of thromboembolism.[30] PDL at the disc of the Amulet device may be compensated by the distal lobe sealing off the appendage. Korsholm and colleagues performed both CCTA and TEE to evaluate PDL at 6 to 8 weeks in 346 patients who received an Amplatzer Cardiac Plug or Amulet device. They found a PDL in 32% of patients with TEE and in 61% of patients with CCTA.[26] A grade 3 PDL (defined as a gap at disc and lobe together with LAA contrast patency) was present in 63 patients (18%) with a discrepancy between modalities in leak quantification. However, PDLs detected with both CCTA and TEE were not significantly associated with worse outcome (hazard ratio: 1.82, 95% confidence interval [CI]: 0.95–3.50; P = .07 and hazard ratio: 1.43, 95% CI: 0.74–2.76; P = .28).[26] In general, CCTA studies have been limited in size and follow-up, so association to outcomes have been difficult.[11,12] The data currently available do, however, raise the question whether PDL evaluation during follow-up is relevant, yet larger studies are needed to confirm these results and evaluate the novel CCTA-based classification. Examples for PDL on TEE and CCTA for the Watchman, Watchman FLX, and Amulet device are shown in Fig. 1.

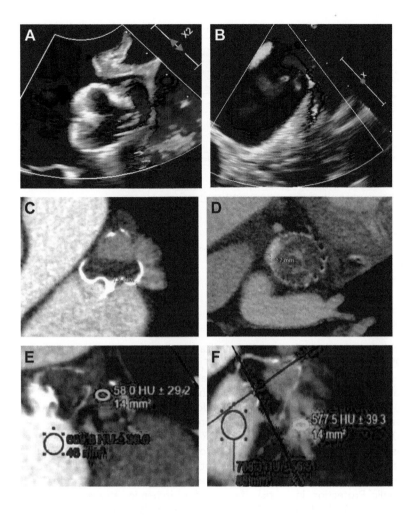

Fig. 1. Examples for peri-device leaks. Peri-device leaks after left atrial appendage closure on TEE with a Watchman device (*A*) and with an Amulet device (*B*), and on CCTA with a Watchman device (*C* and *D*). Linear attenuation coefficient measured in Hounsfield units on CTTA with a Watchman device showing (*E*) complete occlusion of the LAA (no residual contrast patency, 58.0 HU) and (*F*) patent LAA (residual contrast patency, 577.5 HU).

## Management of Peri-Device Leak

In most studies and reviews, the investigators recommended continued oral anticoagulation and serial TEE follow-up for significant PDL.[10,12,13,15,31,32] But this might not be a plausible solution in all patients because LAAO is often performed in patients who cannot accept the long-term oral anticoagulation due to their bleeding diathesis. Therefore, interventional managements to close residual leak have been increasingly performed to reduce the potential risk of the leaks causing thromboembolism. Repeat repositioning of a device during the procedure to decrease the presence of a PDL may not be justified due to the potential increased risk of injury to the LAA, device embolization, or procedure-related pericardial bleeding.[33] However, the placement of a second LAA occluder using an Amplatzer vascular plug may be possible with adequate safety and success, particularly in patients with very large leaks or residual accessory lobes and who are not capable of taking long-term oral anticoagulants.[16,34] Detachable embolization coils are also promising in closing a PDL after LAAO.[35] Preliminary data from the TREASURE (Transcatheter Leak Closure With Detachable Coils Following Incomplete Left Atrial Appendage Closure Procedures) trial (NCT 03503253) showed that detachable coil implantation for residual leaks led to a 92.7% of reduction in leak size, with 93.3% success rate.[10] A suggested algorithm to estimate PDL severity and treatment options is shown in **Fig. 2**.

## Device-Related Thrombus After Percutaneous Device Closure

DRTs has been reported in 1.5% to 14% of patients in association with different occlusion devices.[29,36–40] Fauchier and colleagues[41] found in a retrospective analysis of 469 patients an increased risk of stroke in patients with DRT. A

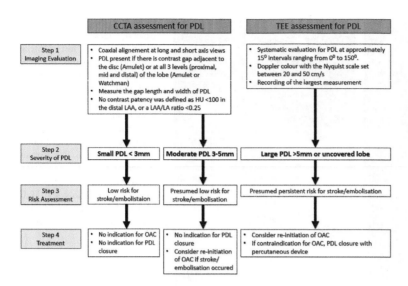

Fig. 2. Suggested algorithm for peri-device leak classification and treatment. Illustration of an algorithm to detect and classify per-device leak (PDL) after left atrial appendage occlusion (LAAO). CCTA, cardiac computed tomography; OAC, oral anticoagulation; TEE, transesophageal echocardiography.

review including 30 studies with 2118 implanted devices reported 82 DRT (3.9%) with a comparable rate among the 3 most common used devices (Watchman and Amplatzer Cardiac Plug/Amulet).[42] A total of 4 (15%) of the 26 patients in whom a thrombus was detected suffered a stroke compared with 3% (10 of 313) of the patients in whom no thrombus was detected. A combined analysis of 4 large and prospective trials, PROTECT-AF (Watchman Left Atrial Appendage System for Embolic Protection in Patients With Atrial Fibrillation) (n = 463); PREVAIL (Evaluation of the Watchman LAA Closure Device in Patients With Atrial Fibrillation vs Long Term Warfarin Therapy) (n = 269); CAP (Continued Access to PROTECT AF registry) (n = 566); and CAP2 (Continued Access to PREVAIL registry) (n = 578), found 65/1739 (3.7%) DRT during a 12-month follow-up period with TEE.[43] DRT was associated with a greater than 3-fold higher risk of stroke and systemic embolism. Concerning the time course, it is not clear when DRTs tend to occur, as patients are mostly asymptomatic and follow-up intervals vary between studies. The Pinnacle FLX study reported DRT in 7 (3.7%) patients after 12 months of follow-up, of whom only 2 of these patients had an embolic event.[28] Dukkipati and colleagues[43] reported that greater than 80% of DRTs occurred later than 45 days after LAAO. DRT was detected in 0.8% (13 of 1706) patients at 45 days, in 1.7% (12 of 692) at 6 months, and in 1.8% (27 of 1504) at 12 months. Late DRTs (>1 year) have been reported but the incidence is unclear and may be due to delayed device endothelialization. Despite the potential occurrence of DRT, event rates after LAAO are overall low both in randomized studies and in large registries, which supports the effectiveness of LAAO. In addition, it must be noted that not each LAA thrombus causes a stroke as well as not each DRT causes a stroke. On the other hand, most of the strokes after LAAO (almost 90%) are not related to DRTs.[44] Instead, they occur in patients who generally have additional risk factors for ischemic stroke without a DRT.[29,36,45–47] The CHA2DS2-VASc score to predict the risk of ischemic stroke and subsequently guide oral anticoagulation use in patients with AF is solely based on clinical risk factors that are also known to increase the risk of stroke in-patients without AF.[48] A meta-analysis including about 600,000 patients revealed that the discrimination ability of the CHA2DS2-VASc risk score was not different among patients with or without nonvalvular AF, suggesting that the risk of stroke is more based on the combination of cardiovascular risk factors and vascular and structural cardiac abnormalities that accompany AF.[49] Therefore, LAAO might only reduce the excess stroke risk attributable to LAA thrombus, a proportion of the excess stroke risk of AF. Strokes after LAAO might be less disabling because it prevents the formation of a large thrombus in a large structure as the LAA. A meta-analysis including 66 studies with 12,033 patients with sample sizes ranging from 12 to 1739 who received most commonly the Watchman (48%), Amplatzer Cardiac Plug (19%), or Amplatzer Amulet (18%) found a pooled incidence of DRT of 3.8% (351 of 10,154 who had follow-up imaging). The pooled incidence of ischemic events was 13.2% (37 of 280) among patients with DRT and 3.8% (285 of 7399) among those without DRT (odds ratio: 5.27, 95% CI: 3.66–7.59; $P < .001$).[50] In general, DRT was associated with a 4- to 5-fold increase in ischemic events, whereas there was no statistically significant difference between different devices.[50] The most recently published meta-analysis including 19 studies reported a rate of 4% for DRT.[17] Korsholm and colleagues[18] directly compared CCTA and TEE 8 weeks and 12 months after LAAO in a single-center registry. In 95% of patients, CCTA and TEE were performed on the same day during follow-up. They reported higher rates of DRT with CCTA (15 patients, 6%) as compared with TEE (5 patients, 2%). However, CCTA allows to illustrate also mild hypoattenuated thickening (HAT) on the atrial surface of the LAA closure device, which was then subsequently subclassified into low- (laminar and thickness <3 mm) or high-grade (≥3 mm thick) HAT. Only a high-grade HAT was considered as definitive DRT on CCTA, which resulted in similar rates of DRT for CCTA and TEE (3.6% vs 2%). After 12 months, only 2 patients (1.4%) were detected with DRT, both with CCTA and TEE. A deep device implantation defined as the device disc being positioned at least 10 mm distal to the tip of the left upper pulmonary vein ridge and thereby leaving an LAA remnant seems to be a predictor for HAT.[18] Examples for DRT on TEE and CCTA for the Watchman, Watchman FLX, and Amulet device are shown in **Fig. 3.**

### Management of Hypoattenuated Thickening and Device-Related Thrombus

Korsholm and colleagues proposed a new clinical graduation of HAT for discrimination between definite thrombus and low-grade HAT, which seems to be a benign and transient phenomenon.[18] It seems that low-grade HAT detected at 8 weeks seemed to resolve spontaneously over time, and a few cases with high-grade HAT regressed into low-grade HAT on anticoagulation therapy. The spontaneous resolution may indicate that low-grade HAT represents temporary platelet aggregation and fibrin deposition as an early stage of thrombus formation. Likewise, studies on transcatheter aortic valve implantation have reported analogous results with hypoattenuation of the leaflets visualized by cardiac CT.[51] Hypoattenuation of the leaflets has been interpreted as early, subclinical stages of leaflet thrombosis, whereas it similarly

seems to spontaneously resolve.[52,53] The mechanisms behind the development of high-grade HAT is unknown. However, it might be a continuum of low-grade HAT, exaggerated by slow flow phenomena, exemplified by the higher prevalence of deep device implantations, permanent AF, and congestive heart failure in patients with high-grade HAT.[18] Evidence of DRT should lead to reinitiation of oral anticoagulation or antiplatelet therapy,[41,42] whereas low-grade HAT seems to advocate a conservative approach.[54] A suggested algorithm to differentiate between low-grade HAT and DRT and treatment options is shown in **Fig. 4.**

### Device Embolization

The reported incidence of LAAO device embolization (DE) varies between 0% and 2%.[55] The PROTECT-AF[56] and PREVAIL[57] studies reported a rate of 0.6% and 0.7%, respectively, for the Watchman device similar to other reports published more recently.[22,58–60] The new-generation Watchman FLX device[32,61] seems to have a much lower DE rate (0% in the PINACLE study).[28] The DE incidence for Amplatzer Cardiac Plug seemed to be slightly higher, with registries reporting up to 2%[62]; however, the incidence with the newer generation Amulet device was less common (0.2%), as shown in a large multicenter registry of 1088 implantations.[29] Most of the DE occur during the procedural or periprocedural period, but delayed embolization has been discovered up to 12 months after the procedure.[55] However, suspicion for DE should arise during follow-up if there are new and otherwise unexplained symptoms such as palpitations or clinical signs of heart failure or after a thoracic trauma, especially in the first weeks to months after implantation.

### SUMMARY

Device surveillance is recommended several hours or the day after the procedure with TTE to detect pericardial effusion or device embolization. In addition, routine follow-up imaging is recommended 6 to 12 weeks post-LAAO with either TEE or CCTA, primarily to assess for DRT and PDL. A routine TTE after 12 months should also be considered to look for late device embolization and to assess routine measurements such as atrial sizes and ventricular and valvular function in patients with AF. Another routine TEE or CCTA should only be repeated after 12 months post-LAAO if the patient is at high risk for recurrent DRT. CCTA and TEE are both valuable options for follow-

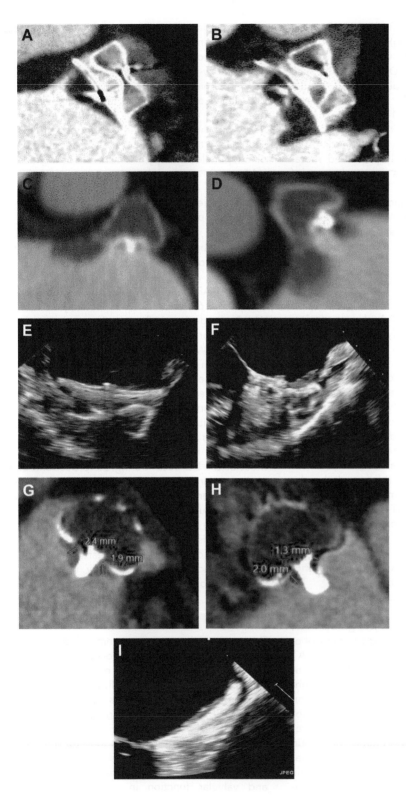

Fig. 3. Examples for hypoatte-nuated thickening and device-related thrombus. Large device-related thrombus after left atrial appendage closure with an Amulet device on CCTA (*A* and *B*) and with a Watchman device (*C* and *D*) and TEE with an Amulet device (*E*) and Watchman device (*F*). Hypoatte-nuated thickening after left atrial appendage closure with a Watchman device on CCTA (*G* and *H*) and on TEE with an Amulet device (*I*).

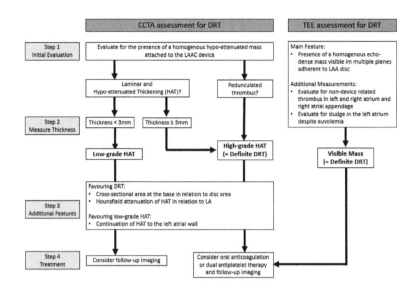

**Fig. 4.** Suggested algorithm for device-related thrombus classification and treatment. Illustration of an algorithm to detect and classify hypoattenuated thickening (HAT) and device-related thrombus (DRT) after left atrial appendage occlusion (LAAO). CCTA, cardiac computed tomography; HU, Hounsfield units; TEE, transesophageal echocardiography.

up imaging after LAAO. TEE is still considered the gold-standard imaging for the LAA in many centers worldwide. CCTA with its high spatial resolution enables comprehensive visualization of the heart both preprocedurally and postprocedurally. The reproducibility is high,[63] and the acquisition allows for postprocessing manipulation of images. Previous studies showed that CCTA provides valuable anatomic information from preprocedural CCTA, which allows prediction of potential challenges during the procedure. However, in the postprocedural setting, the current data on CCTA is still very limited but indicate a superior sensitivity to detect leaks and evaluate device positioning.[19] From a patient perspective, the noninvasive nature, fast acquisition, and nonfasting requirements limit the discomfort. In addition, several potential contraindications and patient's preference against recurrent TEE examinations should be acknowledged. In these cases, CCTA is a good alternative. The associated radiation exposure and subsequent risk should be acknowledged. Also, the risk of contrast-induced nephropathy is a limitation; however, the incidence is low.[20]

To summarize current strategies from the authors' perspective for follow-up imaging, a routine TTE early after the procedure and after 1 year should be performed in all patients. An additional follow-up imaging preferable with CCTA or otherwise with TEE about 6 to 12 weeks post-LAAO is also indicated in most of the patients, especially in all patients in whom the detection of a DRT or large PDL will affect

further treatment strategies. However, a routine follow-up imaging with CCTA or TEE every 6 to 12 months should not be performed and should be restricted to certain patients who suffered from a stroke after LAAO or at high risk for recurrent DRT.

In conclusion, CCTA and TTE are both valuable options during follow-up of LAA closure patients, especially for detecting relevant DRT. CCTA offers superior spatial resolution and imaging of the LAA, leading to a higher sensitivity for detection of residual leaks and evaluation of device positioning. However, further studies are warranted.

## CONFLICT OF INTERESTS

The authors designed the review, gathered, and analyzed relevant randomized trials, registry data, case reports, and device manufacturer information's; wrote the paper; and decided to publish. All authors have read and approved the article. The review has not been published previously and is not being considered for publication elsewhere in whole or in part in any language, including publicly accessible Web sites or e-print servers. Some Figures and Tables were modified and reproduced with permission from the respective journal. We disclose that Dr T. Nestelberger has received research support from the Swiss National Science Foundation (P400PM_191037/1), the Swiss Heart Foundation (FF20079), the Professor Dr Max Cloëtta Foundation, the Margarete und Walter Lichtenstein-Stiftung (3MS1038), the University Basel and the University Hospital Basel as well as speaker honoraria/consulting honoraria from Siemens, Beckman Coulter, Bayer, Ortho Clinical Diagnostics and Orion Pharma, all outside the submitted work. Dr J. Saw has received unrestricted research grant supports (from the Canadian Institutes of Health Research, Heart & Stroke Foundation of Canada, National Institutes of Health, University of British Columbia Division of Cardiology, AstraZeneca, Abbott Vascular, St. Jude Medical, Boston Scientific, and Servier), salary support (Michael Smith Foundation for Health Research), speaker honoraria (AstraZeneca, Abbott Vascular, Boston Scientific, and Sunovion), consultancy and advisory board honoraria (AstraZeneca, St Jude Medical, Abbott Vascular, Boston Scientific, Baylis, Gore, FEops), and proctorship honoraria (Abbott Vascular, St Jude Medical and Boston Scientific), all outside the submitted work. All other authors declare that they have no conflict of interest with this study.

## REFERENCES

1. Go AS, Hylek EM, Phillips KA, et al. Prevalence of diagnosed atrial fibrillation in adults: national implications for rhythm management and stroke prevention: the AnTicoagulation and Risk Factors in Atrial Fibrillation (ATRIA) Study. JAMA 2001;285: 2370–5.
2. Reiffel JA. Atrial fibrillation and stroke: epidemiology. Am J Med 2014;127:e15–6.
3. Nishimura M, Sab S, Reeves RR, et al. Percutaneous left atrial appendage occlusion in atrial fibrillation patients with a contraindication to oral anticoagulation: a focused review. Europace 2018;20:1412–9.
4. Glikson M, Wolff R, Hindricks G, et al. EHRA/EAPCI expert consensus statement on catheter-based left atrial appendage occlusion – an update. EP Eur 2020;22:184.
5. Saw J, Nielsen-Kudsk JE, Bergmann M, et al. Antithrombotic therapy and device-related thrombosis following endovascular left atrial appendage closure. JACC Cardiovasc Interv 2019;12:1067–76.
6. Ismail TF, Panikker S, Markides V, et al. CT imaging for left atrial appendage closure: a review and pictorial essay. J Cardiovasc Comput Tomogr 2015;9:89–102.
7. Ho SY, Cabrera JA, Sanchez-Quintana D. Left Atrial Anatomy Revisited. Circ Arrhythmia Electrophysiol 2012;5:220–8.
8. Wang Y, Di Biase L, Horton RP, et al. Left Atrial Appendage studied by computed tomography to help planning for appendage closure device placement. J Cardiovasc Electrophysiol 2010;21:973–82.
9. Di Biase L, Santangeli P, Anselmino M, et al. Does the left atrial appendage morphology correlate with the risk of stroke in patients with atrial fibrillation? J Am Coll Cardiol 2012;60:531–8.
10. Jang S-J, Wong SC, Mosadegh B. Leaks after left atrial appendage closure: ignored or neglected? Cardiology 2021;146:384–91.
11. Hahn RT, Abraham T, Adams MS, et al. Guidelines for performing a comprehensive transesophageal echocardiographic examination: recommendations from the American Society of Echocardiography and the Society of Cardiovascular Anesthesiologists. J Am Soc Echocardiogr 2013;26:921–64.
12. Viles-Gonzalez JF, Kar S, Douglas P, et al. The clinical impact of incomplete left atrial appendage closure with the Watchman Device in patients with atrial fibrillation: a PROTECT AF (Percutaneous Closure of the Left Atrial Appendage Versus Warfarin Therapy for Prevention of Stroke in Patients Wit. J Am Coll Cardiol 2012;59:923–9.
13. Saw J, Tzikas A, Shakir S, et al. Incidence and clinical impact of device-associated thrombus and peri-device leak following left atrial appendage closure with the amplatzer cardiac plug. JACC Cardiovasc Interv 2017;10:391–9.
14. Salizzoni S, D'Onofrio A, Agrifoglio M, et al. Early and mid-term outcomes of 1904 patients undergoing transcatheter balloon-expandable valve implantation in Italy: results from the Italian Transcatheter Balloon-Expandable Valve Implantation Registry (ITER). Eur J Cardiothorac Surg 2016; 50:1139–48.
15. Raphael CE, Friedman PA, Saw J, et al. Residual leaks following percutaneous left atrial appendage occlusion: assessment and management implications. EuroIntervention 2017;13:1218–25.
16. Alkhouli M, Alqahtani F, Kazienko B, et al. Percutaneous Closure of peridevice leak after left atrial appendage occlusion. JACC Cardiovasc Interv 2018;11:e83–5.
17. Banga S, Osman M, Sengupta PP, et al. CT assessment of the left atrial appendage post-transcatheter occlusion – a systematic review and meta analysis. J Cardiovasc Comput Tomogr 2021;15(4):348–55.
18. Korsholm K, Jensen JM, Nørgaard BL, et al. Detection of device-related thrombosis following left atrial appendage occlusion. Circ Cardiovasc Interv 2019;12(9):e008112.
19. Saw J, Fahmy P, DeJong P, et al. Cardiac CT angiography for device surveillance after endovascular left atrial appendage closure. Eur Hear J – Cardiovasc Imaging 2015;16:1198–206.
20. Korsholm K, Jensen JM, Nielsen-Kudsk JE. Cardiac computed tomography for left atrial appendage occlusion. Interv Cardiol Clin 2018;7:229–42.
21. Romero J, Husain SA, Kelesidis I, et al. Detection of left atrial appendage thrombus by cardiac

computed tomography in patients with atrial fibrillation. Circ Cardiovasc Imaging 2013;6:185–94.

22. Saw J, Lempereur M. Percutaneous left atrial appendage closure: procedural techniques and outcomes. JACC Cardiovasc Interv 2014;7:1205–20.

23. Qamar SR, Jalal S, Nicolaou S, et al. Comparison of cardiac computed tomography angiography and transoesophageal echocardiography for device surveillance after left atrial appendage closure. EuroIntervention 2019;15:663–70.

24. Su P, McCarthy KP, Ho SY. Occluding the left atrial appendage: anatomical considerations. Heart 2008;94:1166–70.

25. Nguyen A, Gallet R, Riant E, et al. Peridevice leak after left atrial appendage closure: incidence, risk factors, and clinical impact. Can J Cardiol 2019; 35:405–12.

26. Korsholm K, Jensen JM, Nørgaard BL, et al. Peridevice leak following amplatzer left atrial appendage occlusion. JACC Cardiovasc Interv 2021;14:83–93.

27. Boersma LVA, Schmidt B, Betts TR, et al. Implant success and safety of left atrial appendage closure with the WATCHMAN device: peri-procedural outcomes from the EWOLUTION registry. Eur Heart J 2016;37:2465–74.

28. Kar S, Doshi SK, Sadhu A, et al. Primary outcome evaluation of a next generation left atrial appendage closure device: results from the PINNACLE FLX Trial. Circulation 2021;143(18):1754–62.

29. Tzikas A, Shakir S, Gafoor S, et al. Left atrial appendage occlusion for stroke prevention in atrial fibrillation: multicentre experience with the AMPLATZER Cardiac Plug. EuroIntervention 2016; 11:1170–9.

30. Kleinecke C, Gloekler S, Meier B. Utilization of percutaneous left atrial appendage closure in patients with atrial fibrillation: an update on patient outcomes. Expert Rev Cardiovasc Ther 2020;18: 517–30.

31. Asmarats L, Rodés-Cabau J. Percutaneous Left Atrial Appendage Closure. Circ Cardiovasc Interv 2017;10(11):e005359.

32. Cruz-Gonzalez I, Korsholm K, Trejo-Velasco B, et al. Procedural and Short-Term Results With the New Watchman FLX Left Atrial Appendage Occlusion Device. JACC Cardiovasc Interv 2020; 13(23):2732–41.

33. Wolfrum M, Attinger-Toller A, Shakir S, et al. Percutaneous left atrial appendage occlusion: Effect of device positioning on outcome. Catheter Cardiovasc Interv 2016;88:656–64.

34. Alkhouli M, Chaker Z, Al-Hajji M, et al. Management of peridevice leak following left atrial appendage occlusion. JACC Clin Electrophysiol 2018;4:967–9.

35. Della Rocca DG, Horton RP, Di Biase L, et al. first experience of transcatheter leak occlusion with

detachable coils following left atrial appendage closure. JACC Cardiovasc Interv 2020;13:306–19.

36. Landmesser U, Tondo C, Camm J, et al. Left atrial appendage occlusion with the AMPLATZER Amulet device: one-year follow-up from the prospective global Amulet observational registry. EuroIntervention 2018;14:e590–7.

37. Holmes DR, Reddy VY, Turi ZG, et al. Percutaneous closure of the left atrial appendage versus warfarin therapy for prevention of stroke in patients with atrial fibrillation: a randomised non-inferiority trial. Lancet (London, England) 2009;374:534–42.

38. Sick PB, Schuler G, Hauptmann KE, et al. Initial worldwide experience with the WATCHMAN left atrial appendage system for stroke prevention in atrial fibrillation. J Am Coll Cardiol 2007;49: 1490–5.

39. Gloekler S, Shakir S, Doblies J, et al. Early results of first versus second generation Amplatzer occluders for left atrial appendage closure in patients with atrial fibrillation. Clin Res Cardiol 2015;104:656–65.

40. Lakkireddy D, Vallakati A, Kanmanthareddy A, et al. Left atrial thrombus formation after successful left atrial appendage ligation: case series from a nationwide survey. J Am Coll Cardiol 2015;65: 1595–6.

41. Fauchier L, Cinaud A, Brigadeau F, et al. Device-related thrombosis after percutaneous left atrial appendage occlusion for atrial fibrillation. J Am Coll Cardiol 2018;71:1528–36.

42. Lempereur M, Aminian A, Freixa X, et al. Device-associated thrombus formation after left atrial appendage occlusion: A systematic review of events reported with the Watchman, the Amplatzer Cardiac Plug and the Amulet. Catheter Cardiovasc Interv 2017;90:E111–21.

43. Dukkipati SR, Kar S, Holmes DR, et al. Device-related thrombus after left atrial appendage closure: incidence, predictors, and outcomes. Circulation 2018;138:874–85.

44. Wunderlich NC, Lorch GC, Honold J, et al. Why follow-up examinations after left atrial appendage closure are important: detection of complications during follow-up and how to deal with them. Curr Cardiol Rep 2020;22:113.

45. Reddy VY, Doshi SK, Kar S, et al. 5-Year outcomes after left atrial appendage closure: from the PREVAIL and PROTECT AF Trials. J Am Coll Cardiol 2017;70:2964–75.

46. Bergmann MW, Ince H, Kische S, et al. Real-world safety and efficacy of WATCHMAN LAA closure at one year in patients on dual antiplatelet therapy: results of the DAPT subgroup from the EWOLUTION all-comers study. EuroIntervention 2018;13: 2003–11.

47. Reddy VY, Gibson DN, Kar S, et al. Post-Approval U.S. experience with left atrial appendage closure

for stroke prevention in atrial fibrillation. J Am Coll Cardiol 2017;69:253–61.

48. Hindricks G, Potpara T, Dagres N, et al. 2020 ESC Guidelines for the diagnosis and management of atrial fibrillation developed in collaboration with the European Association for Cardio-Thoracic Surgery (EACTS). Eur Heart J 2021;42:373–498.

49. Siddiqi TJ, Usman MS, Shahid I, et al. Utility of the CHA2DS2-VASc score for predicting ischaemic stroke in patients with or without atrial fibrillation: a systematic review and meta-analysis. Eur J Prev Cardiol 2021. https://doi.org/10.1093/eurjpc/zwab018.

50. Alkhouli M, Busu T, Shah K, et al. Incidence and Clinical Impact of Device-Related Thrombus Following Percutaneous Left Atrial Appendage Occlusion. JACC Clin Electrophysiol 2018;4:1629–37.

51. Leetmaa T, Hansson NC, Leipsic J, et al. Early aortic transcatheter heart valve thrombosis. Circ Cardiovasc Interv 2015;8(4):e001596.

52. Hansson NC, Grove EL, Andersen HR, et al. Transcatheter aortic valve thrombosis. J Am Coll Cardiol 2016;68:2059–69.

53. Sondergaard L, De Backer O, Kofoed KF, et al. Natural history of subclinical leaflet thrombosis affecting motion in bioprosthetic aortic valves. Eur Heart J 2017;38:2201–7.

54. Cochet H, Iriart X, Sridi S, et al. Left atrial appendage patency and device-related thrombus after percutaneous left atrial appendage occlusion: a computed tomography study. Eur Hear J - Cardiovasc Imaging 2018;19:1351–61.

55. Alkhouli M, Sievert H, Rihal CS. Device embolization in structural heart interventions: incidence, outcomes, and retrieval techniques. JACC Cardiovasc Interv 2019;12:113–26.

56. Reddy VY, Sievert H, Halperin J, et al. Percutaneous left atrial appendage closure vs warfarin for atrial fibrillation: a randomized clinical trial. JAMA 2014; 312:1988–98.

57. Holmes DR, Kar S, Price MJ, et al. Prospective randomized evaluation of the watchman left atrial appendage closure device in patients with atrial fibrillation versus long-term warfarin therapy: the PREVAIL trial. J Am Coll Cardiol 2014;64:1–12.

58. Jazayeri M-A, Vuddanda V, Turagam MK, et al. Safety profiles of percutaneous left atrial appendage closure devices: An analysis of the Food and Drug Administration Manufacturer and User Facility Device Experience (MAUDE) database from 2009 to 2016. J Cardiovasc Electrophysiol 2018;29:5–13.

59. Freeman JV, Varosy P, Price MJ, et al. The NCDR left atrial appendage occlusion registry. J Am Coll Cardiol 2020;75:1503–18.

60. Reddy VY, Möbius-Winkler S, Miller MA, et al. Left atrial appendage closure with the Watchman device in patients with a contraindication for oral anticoagulation: the ASAP study (ASA Plavix Feasibility Study With Watchman Left Atrial Appendage Closure Technology). J Am Coll Cardiol 2013;61: 2551–6.

61. Korsholm K, Samaras A, Andersen A, et al. The Watchman FLX Device. JACC Clin Electrophysiol 2020;6(13):1633–42.

62. Aminian A, Lalmand J, Tzikas A, et al. Embolization of left atrial appendage closure devices: A systematic review of cases reported with the watchman device and the amplatzer cardiac plug. Catheter Cardiovasc Interv 2015;86:128–35.

63. Bai W, Chen Z, Tang H, et al. Assessment of the left atrial appendage structure and morphology: comparison of real-time three-dimensional transesophageal echocardiography and computed tomography. Int J Cardiovasc Imaging 2017;33: 623–33.

# Left Atrial Appendage Closure

## What the Evidence Does and Does Not Reveal—A View from the Outside

Karan Saraf, MBChB, MRCP[a,b],
Gwilym M. Morris, BMBCh, PhD[a,b,*]

---

**KEYWORDS**

- Left atrial appendage closure • Occlusion • Atrial fibrillation

---

**KEY POINTS**

- Left atrial appendage closure (LAAC) with Watchman is inferior to warfarin for ischemic stroke reduction based on randomized data, driven by procedure-related stroke. This complication has reduced in frequency in subsequent nonrandomized registries, but remains uncorroborated by randomized controlled trials (RCTs)
- RCTs in warfarin-eligible cohorts show LAAC with Watchman reduces hemorrhagic stroke, which results in a mortality benefit versus warfarin
- Registry data suggest LAAC is safe and effective for stroke reduction in high bleeding risk/OAC-ineligible AF patients, but ongoing trials are needed versus DOACs before recommendations can be made for widespread adoption in the OAC-eligible population

---

**Abbreviations**

| | |
|---|---|
| SSE | Stroke and Systemic Embolis |
| DRT | Device Related Thrombus |
| OAC | Oral Anti-coagulant |

---

## INTRODUCTION

It is well established that patients with atrial fibrillation (AF) have a significantly increased risk of stroke and systemic embolism (SSE). Treatment with oral anticoagulation (OAC) reduces the risk of SSE in appropriately selected patients to a sufficient degree to offset any increase in bleeding risk conferred by anticoagulation. Warfarin has demonstrated a reduction in SSE of 64%,[1] but in contemporary practice, for most OAC-eligible patients, the current standard of care is treatment with direct oral anticoagulants (DOACs); these have shown at least noninferiority to warfarin in SSE prophylaxis.[2–6] Despite advances in the safety and effectiveness of catheter ablation for AF, improvements in the success of rhythm control have not translated into a reduction in the risk of SSE.[7]

Interest has grown in left atrial appendage closure (LAAC) as a catheter-based therapy with the aim of replacing OAC. If successful, these devices would lead to improved quality of life for patients with AF through reduced medication burden, and removal of lifestyle restrictions due

[a] Division of Cardiovascular Sciences, The University of Manchester, Oxford Road, Manchester M139PL, UK;
[b] Manchester Heart Centre, Manchester University NHS Foundation Trust, Oxford Road, Manchester M139WL, UK
* Corresponding author.
E-mail address: gwilym.morris@manchester.ac.uk

Intervent Cardiol Clin 11 (2022) 171–183
https://doi.org/10.1016/j.iccl.2021.11.009
2211-7458/22/© 2021 Elsevier Inc. All rights reserved.

to bleeding risks of OAC. Furthermore, validated treatment options are needed for OAC-ineligible AF patients who remain at risk of SSE. The current state of evidence for LAAC implantation incites controversy and attracts strong views from both sides of the argument. Most tertiary cardiac centers in the United Kingdom, like ours, perform a high volume of AF ablation, but are not commissioned by the National Health Service to implant LAAC devices; here we present a view of the evidence regarding LAAC, as specialists treating AF but "from the outside" of the LAAC implanter community.

### LAAC—Surgical, Percutaneous or Not At All?

Left atrial appendage (LAA) thrombus has been identified as the source of AF-related strokes in greater than 90% of cases, and thrombus has been observed in the LAA in 27% of all-comers with untreated AF.[8,9] For a detailed discussion of this topic, see the review by Cresti and Camara in this journal issue. Initial attempts to exclude the LAA were via a direct surgical approach usually concurrent to other cardiac surgery for patients thought to be at increased risk of stroke. Despite the apparent attractiveness of this approach both the American Heart Association (AHA)/American College of Cardiology (ACC)/Heart Rhythm Society (HRS) and the European Society of Cardiology (ESC) guidelines state surgical closure of the LAA should be considered only in patients with AF who are undergoing cardiac surgery for another reason (class IIb, level of evidence B), and importantly, even in the presence of apparent successful surgical closure, OAC should be continued indefinitely.[10,11]

The risk/benefit assessment of surgical LAAC is clouded by potential increases in postoperative complications, incomplete appendage closure (19%–59%), thrombus formation in the remaining stump (25%), and subsequent embolic events (2.6%–8%).[12–14] Nuanced interpretation is made more difficult by the confounding effect of the concomitant surgery performed in published trials (eg, bypass and/or valve surgery), but perhaps most importantly a variety of methods used to exclude the LAA, including sutures, staples, or epicardial closure devices.[12]

The LAAOS III trial, published in May 2021, appears to have provided a robust response to previously unanswered questions regarding the efficacy and safety of surgical LAAC. A total of 4770 patients with AF and CHA$_2$DS$_2$VASc $\geq$2 undergoing cardiac surgery for another indication were randomized to receive concomitant surgical LAAC or no LAAC. At 3.8 years follow-up, SSE occurred in 4.8% in the LAAC group versus 7.0% in the standard care group (31% relative risk reduction [RRR], $P$ = .001), with no difference in periprocedural adverse events or all-cause mortality between groups. This benefit was achieved despite similar numbers of patients in both groups continuing with long-term OAC.[15]

### IS PERCUTANEOUS LAAC A BETTER OPTION?

Although LAAOS III may shape future practice for concomitant LAAC in patients undergoing cardiac surgery, in most AF patients who do not have a surgical indication, there are potential advantages to a percutaneous approach. Treatment for stroke prophylaxis in AF patients remains imperfect; anticoagulation confers a significant bleeding risk, excluding it as a therapy for patients with an elevated risk of hemorrhage. A safe and effective percutaneous therapy that reduced the risk of SSE would bring measurable improvements in mortality, morbidity, and quality of life. Despite these potential advantages, the American and European guidelines agree that percutaneous LAAC should only be considered in patients with contraindications to long-term anticoagulation (life-threatening bleeding or intracranial hemorrhage without treatable cause).[10,11] The position of these guideline committees was that the evidence for percutaneous LAAC in this population is of moderate quality from predominantly non-randomized studies and meta-analyses, resulting in a class IIb/B recommendation.

### What Randomized Trial Data is There?

There are 3 completed randomized controlled trials (RCTs) comparing LAAC to warfarin (PROTECT AF and PREVAIL)[16,17] or DOACs (PRAGUE-17)[18] in OAC-eligible patients (summarized in Table 1).

PROTECT AF (2005–2008) randomized 707 patients with CHADS$_2$ $\geq$1 to LAAC using the first-generation Watchman device (Boston Scientific, Marlborough MA) or warfarin (2:1, respectively).[17] For the primary composite efficacy endpoint of SSE and cardiovascular (CV) death, LAAC achieved noninferiority (probability >0.999) and superiority (probability >0.960) at 5 years (2.3% vs 3.7%/100 patient-years [PY]). This was driven by significant reductions in hemorrhagic stroke (Watchman 0.6% vs warfarin 4%/100PY) and CV death (1% vs 2.4%/100PY). Ischemic stroke

**Table 1**
Summary of randomized controlled trials investigating left atrial appendage closure versus oral anticoagulation

| | Primary Efficacy Endpoints | Primary Safety Endpoints | Other Endpoints |
|---|---|---|---|
| **PROTECT AF[17]** | | | |
| Design<br>2:1 Watchman vs VKA (2005–2009)<br>Bayesian analysis—707 patients<br>Inclusion<br>$CHADS_2 \geq 1$<br>Characteristics<br>VKA TTR = 70%<br>Mean $CHADS_2$ = 2.2,<br>$CHA_2DS_2VASc$ = 3.5<br>Implant success 90.9% | Composite stroke, SE, CV/unexplained death<br>2.3% vs 3.8% events/100PY (40% RRR, 1.5% ARR—NI and superiority achieved) | Composite serious pericardial effusion, stroke, device embolization, major bleeding<br>3.6% vs 3.1% events/100PY (NI achieved)<br>Serious pericardial effusion 4.8%<br>Major bleeding 4.8% vs 7.4%<br>Procedure-related ischemic stroke 1.3% | Ischemic stroke<br>1.4% vs 1.1%/100PY (ns)<br>Hemorrhagic stroke<br>0.6% vs 4%/100PY<br>CV death<br>1% vs 2.4%/100PY (60% RRR, 1.4% ARR vs VKA)<br>All-cause death<br>3.2% vs 4.8% events/100PY (34% RRR, 5.7% ARR vs VKA) |
| **PREVAIL[16]** | **Primary Efficacy Endpoints** | **Primary Safety Endpoints** | **Other Endpoints** |
| Design<br>2:1 Watchman vs VKA (2010–2012)<br>Bayesian analysis—407 patients<br>Inclusion<br>$CHADS_2 \geq 2$<br>Characteristics<br>VKA group TTR = 68%<br>Mean $CHADS_2$ = 2.8,<br>$CHA_2DS_2VASc$ = 4<br>Implant success 95.1% | Composite stroke, SE, CV/unexplained death<br>18-mo event rates 0.066 vs 0.051 (NI not achieved)<br>Composite late ischemic stroke and SE (>7 d postimplant)<br>0.0255 vs 0.0135 (NI achieved) | Early safety of device group—composite all-death, ischemic stroke, SE, device-related complications requiring intervention (excluding pericardiocentesis, snaring of embolized device, nonsurgical access complications)<br>2.2% (success achieved vs performance goal from PROTECT AF) | ALL procedural complications (including serious effusion, perforation, embolization, vascular) 4.2%<br>Embolization 0.7%<br>Cardiac perforation 0.4%<br>Tamponade 0.4%<br>Major bleeding 0.4% |
| **5-y PROTECT AF & PREVAIL Meta-analysis[20]** | **Efficacy Endpoints** | | **Safety Endpoints** |
| Combined patient-level meta-analysis<br>Frequentist analysis<br>Patients with $CHADSVASc \geq 2$ | Composite stroke, SE, CV/unexplained death<br>2.8% vs 3.4%/100PY (P = .27, NI achieved)<br>All stroke/SE | | All major bleeding (including procedural tamponade, vascular complications)<br>3.1% vs 3.5%/100PY (P = .60) |

(continued on next page)

## 5-y PROTECT AF & PREVAIL Meta-analysis[20]

| | Efficacy Endpoints | Safety Endpoints |
|---|---|---|
| PROTECT AF = 93%<br>PREVAIL = 100% | 1.7% vs 1.8%/100PY (P = .87, NI achieved)<br>Disabling stroke<br>0.44% vs 1%/100PY (P = .03)<br>CV death<br>1.3% vs 2.2%/100PY (P = .027)<br>All-cause death<br>3.6% vs 4.9%/100PY (P = .035) | Non-procedure-related major bleeding<br>1.7% vs 3.6% (P = .0003)<br>Hemorrhagic stroke<br>0.17% 0.87%/100PY (P = .0022) |

## PRAGUE-17[18]

| | Primary Endpoints | Safety | Secondary Endpoints |
|---|---|---|---|
| Design<br>1:1 Amulet/Watchman vs DOAC 2015–2019<br>Inclusion<br>bleeding history requiring hospitalization or cardioembolism on OAC or CHADSVASC≥3 & HAS-BLED≥2<br>Characteristics<br>402 patients–mean CHADSVASC 4.7<br>Implant success 96.8% | Composite of safety and efficacy:<br>Stroke or TIA, SE, clinically significant bleeding, CV death, device-related complications<br>10.99% vs 13.42%/100PY (P = .44, NI achieved) | Procedure-related complications<br>4.8% | All stroke<br>2.6% vs 2.57%/y<br>CV death<br>3.18% vs 4.28%/y<br>Major bleeding<br>5.5% vs 7.42%/y<br>Ischemic stroke<br>2.2 vs 2.38%/y |

*Abbreviations:* ARR, absolute risk reduction; CV, cardiovascular; DOAC, direct oral anticoagulant; NI, noninferiority; ns, nonsignificant; OAC, oral anticoagulant; PY, patient-years; RRR, relative risk reduction; SE, systemic embolism; TTR, time in therapeutic range; VKA, vitamin K antagonist.

(1.4% vs 1.1%/100PY) did not reach noninferiority, and although all-cause stroke rates were nonsignificant, there were significantly fewer fatal or disabling strokes with LAAC (0.5% vs 1.2%/100PY). There was also superiority for all-cause mortality (3.2% vs 4.8%/100PY).

For the primary composite safety endpoint of cardiac tamponade, stroke, device embolization, and major bleeding, noninferiority was achieved (2.3% vs 5.8%/100PY, probability 0.980). Individually, major bleeding was 8.9% in the device group versus 7.4% in the warfarin group, procedure-related stroke 2.6%, tamponade 4.8%, and device embolization 0.6%. Device-related events occurred mostly in the 7 days postprocedure, whereas warfarin-related events were distributed linearly over time.

Following PROTECT AF, the United States Food and Drug Administration expressed concern that 31% of patients had a $CHADS_2$ score of only 1, and that there was a high early safety event rate.[17,19] With further investigation mandated, PREVAIL (2010–2012)[16] randomized 407 patients with $CHADS_2 \geq 2$ to Watchman and warfarin (2:1), respectively. In contrast to PROTECT AF, LAAC failed to reach noninferiority for the composite endpoint of SSE or CV death, which may have been due to an unusually low stroke rate in the warfarin arm of 0.73%. This is lower than the warfarin groups in PROTECT AF[17] (1.1%) and the DOAC trials, although patients enrolled in PREVAIL were a higher-risk population than these trials, with a mean $CHA_2DS_2VASc$ score of 4 (stroke in RE-LY 1.2%,[2] ROCKET-AF 1.42%,[5] ARISTOTLE 1.05%,[4] ENGAGE-AF TIMI-48 1.25%[3]). It may be that PREVAIL was underpowered, with small sample size (n = 138 in the warfarin arm) and point estimate of low confidence perhaps contributing toward a reduced ability to establish noninferiority. The authors justified the sample size by having designed PREVAIL only for analysis in combination with PROTECT AF, from which informative priors were borrowed for its Bayesian design.[20,21]

The second coprimary endpoint of ischemic events from 7 days postimplantation looked at device efficacy once already implanted, thus excluding most procedural complications; LAAC was noninferior, suggesting a long-term ischemic event reduction as effective as warfarin, consistent with the mechanistic hypothesis of cardioembolism from the LAA being the main cause of SSE in AF. Lastly, the third composite procedural safety endpoint of 4.2% was considerably lower than in PROTECT AF.[16]

A 5-year combined patient-level meta-analysis of PROTECT AF and PREVAIL showed that overall SSE rates were similar between LAAC and warfarin (1.6% vs 0.95%, $P = .08$), whereas LAAC demonstrated 80% RRR in hemorrhagic stroke (0.17% vs 0.87%, $P = .0022$), and of those strokes which occurred, 55% fewer were disabling or fatal ($P = .03$). LAAC with Watchman resulted in 41% ($P = .027$) and 27% ($P = .035$) RRR in CV and all-cause mortality, respectively (0.9% and 1.3% absolute risk reductions, respectively), driven by hemorrhagic stroke reduction, congruent with the putative basis of mortality reduction also seen with DOACs versus warfarin.

It remains unclear how much the potential benefits of LAAC are offset by procedural complications. Improvements in safety will lower the bar for benefit to be realized. Iterative improvements in device design and procedural expertise have been demonstrated in more recent trials. The accepted definition of successful device implantation is the presence of $\leq 5$ mm peridevice leak (PDL). Small leaks have not been robustly shown to significantly increase rates of SSE.[22] Implantation success improved between PROTECT-AF (90.9%) and PREVAIL (95.1%), whereas overall complications reduced from 8.7% to 4.2%, including reduction in tamponade (4.8% to 1.9%) and device-related stroke (2.6% to 0.4%).[20]

When considering the use of these devices, and the guideline recommendation in warfarin-ineligible patients only, a significant limitation of these studies is that the use of antithrombotic therapy for at least 6 weeks postimplant means that enrolled patients were long-term OAC-eligible. It is therefore difficult to generalize the results to the OAC-ineligible, who may represent a different cohort. The subsequent recommendation in guidelines that only contraindicated patients be considered for LAAC, therefore, applies to patients not represented in the RCTs. Also, the combined mean $CHA_2DS_2$-VASc and HAS-BLED scores were 3.6 and 1.8, respectively, providing information only for a moderate-risk population, and patients were predominantly male and Caucasian. Furthermore, as the DOAC versus warfarin trials revealed reductions in SSE, hemorrhagic stroke, and mortality by 19%, 51%, and 10%, respectively, there has been a transition toward DOACs as first-line OAC in real-world practice, meaning PROTECT AF and PREVAIL data versus warfarin cannot be generalized to contemporary OAC use.[23]

PRAGUE-17 (2015–2019) evaluated LAAC against DOACs to provide an updated comparison in the current era of safer and more effective anticoagulation.[18] A total of 402 patients with $CHA_2DS_2VASc \geq 3$ and HAS-BLED $\geq 2$, or history of serious bleeding or cardioembolism on OAC were enrolled. Mean $CHA_2DS_2VASc$ was 4.7 and HAS-BLED 3, denoting higher-risk patients than PROTECT AF and PREVAIL. Following European practice, the postprocedure antithrombotic regimen consisted of dual antiplatelet therapy (DAPT) with aspirin and clopidogrel for 3 months, followed by aspirin alone. 95.5% of patients in the DOAC arm received apixaban; 61.3%, 35.9%, and 2.8% in the LAAC arm received the Amplatzer Amulet (St Jude Medical, St Paul, MN), Watchman, and Watchman FLX devices, respectively. The primary composite endpoint combined both efficacy and safety outcomes of both treatments: all stroke, SE, major bleeding, CV death, and device-related complications. This occurred in 10.99% and 13.42% of the LAAC and DOAC groups, respectively, achieving noninferiority ($P$ value for noninferiority 0.004). Overall procedural complications occurred in 4.8% (tamponade 1.5%, device embolization 0.5%, bleeding 1%, procedure-related death 1%). There were no statistically significant differences in the secondary endpoints of stroke, bleeding and CV or all-cause mortality.[18]

LAAC met noninferiority margins, and secondary analyses showed individual endpoints were similar between groups, but the trial was considerably underpowered for these analyses. The authors concluded LAAC is noninferior to DOAC, an interpretation that has led to considerable controversy. The combination of efficacy and safety endpoints in noninferiority design means grouping events (SSE and bleeding) that are expected to trend in opposite directions. This favors the experimental therapy by biasing to the null hypothesis, making noninferiority easier to achieve, in addition to creating uncertainty regarding the contribution of individual endpoints to the overall results. More data are required before LAAC can be considered equivalent to DOACs.[24]

## Can We Rely on Nonrandomized Studies and Registries?

Despite the relatively widespread use of percutaneous LAAC, the 3 trials discussed in the previous section are the only randomized data available. Most LAAC implantation outcomes come from registry data, largely focusing on the Watchman device. By necessity, patients enrolled in registries are at higher risk than those in the RCTs, including those with previous bleeding on, or some form of contraindication to OAC, because this is what the guidelines recommend.

A 2018 meta-analysis by Baman and colleagues aggregated 15 LAAC registries[25]; the larger studies (n > 150) from this meta-analysis, as well as the NCDR registry and PINNACLE FLX, published in 2020 after the meta-analysis, and cumulative data are presented in Table 2.[25,26] We can gain "real-world" insight into procedural success and complications from these data. Implantation success rates ranged between 94.2% and 98.8% across all devices (Watchman, Amplatzer, and Lariat [SentreHEART, Redwood City, CA]). Comparing Watchman data with PROTECT AF and PREVAIL, mean success rates appear to have improved from ~92% to 98%. Complications appear to decline over time as compared with initial experience. Pericardial effusion remained consistently the most common, from 4.8% and 1.9% in PROTECT AF and PREVAIL to 1.4% across registries. Major bleeding (1.3%), device embolization (0.09%), procedure-related stroke (0.15%), and death (0.17%) were similarly low. In registries reporting efficacy outcomes, ischemic stroke occurred in 0.9% to 1.7% and all-cause mortality in up to 5%, demonstrating the high-risk population in these data sets.[25,26]

Although important that focus remains on RCT data for safety and efficacy outcomes, we can perhaps look to registries and nonrandomized data to learn more about contemporary improvements in procedural success and reductions in complications, especially from the use of devices in smaller centers outside of trials. Improvements in implant techniques and device technology may be able to drive down complication rates and improve implantation success sufficiently to result in wider acceptance if these can be demonstrated in future RCTs. The NCDR is a North American postapproval registry evaluating all US Watchman implants since 2016, it is the largest registry by some margin including 38,158 patients at last report.[26] Implantation success was high at 98.3% and in-hospital adverse events considerably lower than PROTECT AF and PREVAIL (tamponade 1.39%, major bleeding 1.4%, device embolization 0.07%, procedure-related stroke 0.16%, death 0.19%; Table 2). This registry includes smaller centers and lower volume operators with the median implants per operator being 12.[25,26]

Other important devices not represented in published RCTs are the Watchman FLX,

**Table 2**
Summary of registry and nonrandomized trials investigating left atrial appendage closure

| Major registries[25-27] (n ≥ 150) | Device/success rate | Long-Term Outcomes | | | Procedural Complications/Safety Outcomes | | | | |
|---|---|---|---|---|---|---|---|---|---|
| | | Ischemic stroke | Hemorrhagic stroke | All-cause mortality | Pericardial effusion ± tamponade | Major bleeding | Device embolization | Procedure-related stroke/TIA | Procedure-related death |
| CAP 2008–2010 n = 460 | Watchman/95% | NR | NR | NR | 2.2% | 0.7% | 0% | 0% | 0% |
| ASAP 2009–2011 n = 150 | Watchman/94.7% | 1.7% | 0.6% | 5% | 3.3% | 1.3% | 1.3% | 0.7% | 0% |
| CAP2 2012–2014 n = 579 | Watchman/94.8% | NR | NR | NR | 2.4% | NR | 0% | 0.35% | 0% |
| EWOLUTION 2013–2015 n = 1021 | Watchman/98.5% | 0.3% | 0% | 0.7% | 0.5% | 0.7% | 0.2% | NR | 0% |
| US Post-Approval 2015–2016 n = 3822 | Watchman/95.6% | NR | NR | NR | 1.3% | NR | 0.2% | 0.08% | 0.08% |
| NCDR 2016–2018 n = 38,158 | Watchman/98.3% | NR | NR | NR | 1.39% | 1.25% | 0.07% | 0.16% | 0.19% |
| PINNACLE FLX 2018 N = 400 | Watchman FLX/98.8% | NR | NR | NR | 1% | NR | 0% | 0.5% | 0% |
| Tzikas et al 2008–2013 n = 1047 | ACP/97.3% | Composite stroke 0.9% | | 4.3% | 1.4% | 1.3% | 1% | 0.9% | 0.8% |
| Koskinas et al 2009–2014 n = 500 | ACP/Amulet/97.8% | NR | NR | NR | 6.6% | 3.4% | 2% | 1% | 0.4% |
| Price et al 2014 n = 154 | Lariat/94.2% | Composite stroke 1.3% | | 1.9% | 10.3% | 9.1% | N/A | 0% | 0.6% |
| Lakkireddy et al 2016 n = 712 | Lariat/95.5% | NR | NR | NR | NR | 0% | N/A | 0% | 0.1% |
| **Cumulative safety/procedural outcomes by device (all registries)[25-27]** | | | | | Pericardial effusion ± tamponade | Major bleeding | Device embolization | Procedure-related stroke | Procedure-related death |
| Watchman n = 44,190 | 98% | | | | 1.4% | 1.3% | 0.09% | 0.15% | 0.17% |
| Amplatzer ACP/Amulet n = 1266 | 97% | | | | 1.3% | 1.2% | 1% | 0.7% | 0.66% |
| Lariat n = 955 | 95.3% | | | | 6.5% | 1.5% | N/A | 0% | 0.17% |

Abbreviations: NR, not reported; N/A, not applicable.

Amplatzer ACP and Amulet, and Lariat devices. The nonrandomized PINNACLE FLX study evaluated the next-generation Watchman FLX device, which was designed to improve on the previous generation Watchman to reduce tamponade, embolization, and periprocedural stroke. A total of 400 patients with a mean $CHA_2DS_2VASc$ of $4.2 \pm 1.5$ and HAS-BLED $2.0 \pm 1.0$ were enrolled. Implant success was 98.8%. One-year safety events showed 1% tamponade, 0.5% procedure-related stroke, with no reported device embolizations, and no procedure-related deaths.[27]

Registry data suggest that Amplatzer devices have similar success rates and outcomes to those seen with Watchman (97%); tamponade and major bleeding events occurred in 1.3% and 1.2%, respectively. Mean $CHA_2DS_2VASc$ was 4.5 and HAS-BLED 3.1.[25] The Lariat device, a hybrid epicardial-endocardial device, has shown lower implantation success of 94%. There are concerns about the safety of the Lariat, with a 7.5% tamponade rate as well as a 3.4% occurrence (24 patients) of LAA laceration, with 10 patients requiring surgical repair.[25,28]

Further details on the different devices are covered in this series.

## HOW SHOULD THE DATA SHAPE OUR PRACTICE?

### Early Outcomes

There are valid criticisms of all LAAC techniques regarding procedural safety. A new intervention cannot be considered an alternative to the current gold standard if it results in a greater burden of serious adverse events. Procedural complications have reduced over time (PROTECT AF 8.7%, PREVAIL 4.5%, CAP 2.9%, and PINNACLE FLX 1.5%).[25,27] This is attributed to increased operator experience and education, improved preprocedural planning using computed tomography (CT), and patient selection. The overall serious complication rate across all randomized and nonrandomized Watchman studies is 3% to 3.5%. However, it is important to note that the more contemporary data come from registries, which are prone to bias from under-reporting and a lack of independent event adjudication, especially for safety events, so in the absence of corroborating RCTs, registry data must be interpreted with caution. There are data to suggest that major procedural complications are significantly reduced in higher volume (n ≥ 32 implants/y) versus lower volume centers (odds ratio 0.55, $P = .003$).[29] This is significantly higher than the median 12 implants/y seen in the NCDR registry, suggesting

a learning curve to be navigated for operators and institutions, but provides hope that procedural safety can improve with greater operator experience.

Indeed, proponents argue that as complications reduce further, LAAC cannot be considered riskier than some other invasive cardiac procedures, such as AF ablation. Systematic reviews estimate periprocedural complications from contemporary AF ablation at 3.5% to 4%.[30] Major adverse events from transcatheter aortic valve replacement (TAVR) are up to 20%[31] and permanent pacemaker (PPM) implantation complications 4% to 8%.[32] However, TAVR and PPMs offer prognostic benefit with no medication alternatives for their respective indications,[31,33] and AF ablation has been shown to be superior to medical therapy for rhythm control,[34] therefore directly comparing their complication rates and those of LAAC is of limited use.

### Longer-Term Outcomes

Randomized data show higher annualized ischemic stroke with Watchman than OAC. These are mostly procedure-related; from a mechanistic perspective, once the LAA was closed, stroke rates were equivalent at 1.1% each.[20] With time, procedure-related stroke has reduced from 1.3% in PROTECT AF to a mean of 0.15% in nonrandomized registries (though we have noted the limitations of registries). Furthermore, ischemic stroke severity appears reduced with LAAC (56% fewer disabling or fatal strokes in PROTECT AF).[20,21,25]

The Watchman device was associated with significant reductions in hemorrhagic stroke, CV and all-cause death in the RCTs. Hemorrhagic stroke often results in greater disability or death than ischemic stroke, and therefore it could be argued that LAAC not only provides some overall reduction in ischemic stroke (albeit inferior to warfarin) but also without the bleeding associated with the latter, resulting in a mortality benefit.[21,25,26,35]

### What Questions Remain Unanswered?

Although LAAC is positioned as noninferior to warfarin, the latter has largely been superseded by DOACs, themselves having robustly proven at least noninferiority in stroke reduction, and superiority in bleeding and mortality.[2–5] There are no data allowing us to draw a direct conclusion about the efficacy of LAAC versus DOACs; the mixed composite trial design of PRAGUE-17 prevents accurate comparison for either efficacy or safety. This calls into question the

**Table 3**
Current in-progress randomized clinical trials investigating left atrial appendage closure

| Study | N | Description | Expected Completion |
|---|---|---|---|
| CLOSURE-AF | 1512 | LAAC (any approved device) vs DOAC | 2021 |
| CATALYST | 2650 | Amplatzer Amulet vs DOAC | 2024 |
| OPTION | 1600 | Watchman FLX vs OAC | 2024 |
| OCCLUSION-AF | 750 | LAAC (any approved device) vs DOAC | 2024 |
| CHAMPION-AF | 3000 | Watchman FLX vs DOAC | 2025 |

*Abbreviations:* AF, atrial fibrillation; DOAC, direct oral anticoagulant; LAAC, left atrial appendage closure; OAC, oral anticoagulant.

proposal that LAAC could be considered a direct alternative to DOACs in long-term OAC-eligible patients, if much of the potential benefit of LAAC is driven by a reduction in hemorrhage compared with warfarin this may not be maintained against DOACS where the bleeding risk is substantially lower. Several RCTs comparing LAAC with DOACs are currently in progress (**Table 3**).[18,23,35]

The optimum postprocedural anticoagulation and antiplatelet regimen remain unknown. PROTECT AF and PREVAIL used warfarin and aspirin for 45 days. At this point, if transesophageal echocardiogram (TEE) demonstrated no device-related thrombus (DRT) or PDL >5 mm, warfarin was replaced with clopidogrel and DAPT continued for 6 months, followed by aspirin alone. This regimen is standard in the United States, whereas Europe has largely opted for DAPT (aspirin and clopidogrel) up to 3 months, followed by aspirin only.[16,17,36]

Short-term DAPT potentially offers reduced overall bleeding compared with OAC, but may result in increased thrombus formation. Analysis of patients in the EWOLUTION registry who received follow-up TEE or CT (n = 835, median 54 days) revealed 4.1% DRT (2.4% on OAC, 4.7% DAPT, 2.0% no treatment; $P = .16$). Differences between treatments were statistically nonsignificant, suggesting other factors may have played a part in thrombogenesis, potentially the LAA ostium diameter, and therefore device size.[37] The bleeding events were also not significantly different between groups.[36,37]

Søndergaard and colleagues reported a propensity-matched retrospective comparison of 1527 Watchman patients receiving OAC or APT postprocedure. Nonprocedural bleeding (OAC 4.3% vs APT 4.5%, $P = .775$) and thromboembolism (OAC 1.2% vs APT 0.6%, $P = .089$) were similar; however, DRT occurred more frequently in the APT group (3.1% vs OAC 1.4%, $P = .018$).[38] In summary, current data have not robustly identified the optimum postprocedure pharmacologic strategy. This presents challenges, as the long-term reduction in hemorrhagic stroke associated with LAAC has to be weighed up against the short-term bleeding risk with APT/OAC in the already high bleeding risk cohort undergoing this intervention, together with DRT risk in those not on OAC.

Further complicating decisions around peri-procedural management are a paucity of robust randomized evidence for the management of patients with contraindications to OAC. Only patients with a "previous life-threatening bleed without reversible cause" are recommended for LAAC by American and European guidelines. The definition of "contraindication" in real-world practice varies, and there is often overlap with those considered high-risk. For example, 47.8% of patients in PRAGUE-17 experienced prior major bleeding events; a proportion of these would be considered contraindicated as per the guideline definition, though were enrolled due to being "high risk."[18] The only data available in this cohort arises from mostly small nonrandomized studies, as recruiting truly contraindicated patients prospectively has been extremely difficult, as evidenced by the recent closing of the ASAP-TOO trial (clinical trial NCT02928497) due to inadequate enrollment. It may be difficult for physicians to justify enrolling a truly OAC-contraindicated patient with no option but LAAC into an RCT with a chance of randomization to either APT or no treatment, either of which may be unacceptable because of high bleeding risk, or high thromboembolic risk, respectively.[10,11]

A 2021 meta-analysis of 7951 patients by Labori and colleagues evaluated outcomes from LAAC in OAC-ineligible patients. Mean $CHA_2DS_2VASc$ and HAS-BLED scores were 4.32 and 3.19, respectively, and mean follow-up 1.46 years. 37.5% previously had a stroke and 60.3% major bleeding. The majority received DAPT for 1 to 6 months postprocedure, followed by aspirin only.[39] Ischemic stroke after LAAC was 1.39/100PY compared with the predicted rate of 5.5/100PY, a 74.7% reduction favoring LAAC. Major bleeding events were 2.22/100PY and all-cause death 4.38/100PY.

This event rate in very high-risk patients is similar to the cumulative ischemic event rate in PROTECT AF and PREVAIL (1.3 per 100PY), as well as previously published systematic reviews and meta-analyses.[20,40,41] Bleeding events were also comparable to other studies, suggesting that LAAC may be effective at reducing stroke risk in the absence of OAC in this cohort. Finally, a systematic review of patients with prior intracranial hemorrhage (n = 727, CHA$_2$DS$_2$VASc 4–5.2, HAS-BLED 3–4.7) found rates of ischemic stroke (1.6%) and recurrent intracranial hemorrhage (1.5%) to be low following LAAC. Given the lack of alternative treatment, LAAC in this scenario with short-term postprocedural use of either OAC or DAPT seems reasonable.[42] Although the limitations that usually apply when analyzing non-RCT or observational data should be considered, these types of systematic reviews and meta-analyses remain the best insight available in these cohorts. Given guidelines already support LAAC in these groups, the ensuing recruitment difficulties may make much-desired RCTs unfeasible.

In addition, many patients with LAAC may fall victim to one of the commonest concerns in medicine, navigating between Scylla and Charybdis of high bleeding risk in the presence of intracardiac thrombus. DRT is a significant complication, that undoubtedly contributes to the stroke rate in LAAC trials. DRT may occur because of an incomplete endothelialization, suboptimal device positioning, incomplete LAA occlusion, or antithrombotic nonadherence.[43] A recent meta-analysis of 12,033 patients reported 3.8% incidence of device thrombus on TEE.[44,45] Analysis of DRT in the PROTECT AF and PREVAIL RCTs, and CAP and CAP2 registries found a 4-fold increase in ischemic events (25% of DRT patients suffered ischemic stroke vs 6.8% of non-DRT patients over 7159PY of follow-up).[45] However, three-quarters of DRT patients did not experience SSE, and because DRT was uncommon (3.74%), most events occurred in non-DRT patients (86.6%). There was an association between TEE surveillance frequency in the RCTs and increased DRT detection, as compared with the registries, suggesting that DRT occurs at some point in a larger proportion of patients.

Not all LAA thrombus results in stroke, however, so it is plausible that not all DRT results in stroke, and therefore clinically significant events are not always observed following DRT, which is often detected incidentally following protocol-mandated surveillance.[45]

Clearly, however, DRT is not benign, and its treatment with extended duration therapeutic OAC further increases bleeding risk in an already high-risk cohort who are undergoing an invasive procedure to avoid long-term anticoagulation. It is unclear how long to treat patients with OAC or whether to stop treatment once DRT resolves, as the underlying mechanism resulting in DRT will still be present. Further investigation is also required to determine optimum surveillance frequency, modifiable DRT risk factors, and continuing device and procedural improvements to reduce its incidence.

## DOES THE EVIDENCE SUPPORT THE USE OF LAAC AND ARE THE GUIDELINES CORRECTLY POSITIONED?

Use of the Watchman device is supported by evidence drawn from RCTs. Compared with warfarin, noninferiority for ischemic stroke reduction has not been demonstrated, with superiority for hemorrhagic, disabling and fatal strokes, and mortality.[21,25] The case for routine use is weakened by the lack of data comparing safety and efficacy with DOACs. There are less data for other devices, and different devices have yet to be evaluated in head-to-head studies. Accounting for these gaps in the evidence, the guideline positions that LAAC should only be considered in OAC-ineligible patients seem reasonable. The up-front procedural risk demonstrated in RCT data is currently unacceptable in the OAC-eligible patient who can be treated with a DOAC, although this cohort has not been specifically studied in RCTs. LAAC demonstrated inferiority in ischemic stroke reduction in RCTs, and it is not clear that the benefits driven by bleeding reduction will be maintained when compared to a DOAC rather than warfarin.

If forthcoming RCTs (see Table 3) fail to show at least equivalence in SSE reduction with LAAC compared to DOACs, we wonder whether in the future, a major role for LAAC may be in the patient for whom OAC would be undesirable or contraindicated for the indication of hemorrhagic risk reduction, rather than for SSE reduction. Some of these patient types may already be receiving LAAC, as observed in one meta-analysis, with 60.3% having a previous major hemorrhage.[39] In these patients and those with a disproportionately high bleeding to ischemic risk, where the benefit/risk ratio of OAC is less favorable than the general OAC-eligible population, practice may evolve to pragmatically accept lower ischemic stroke reduction with LAAC, instead favoring significant hemorrhagic risk reduction, especially given that hemorrhagic stroke is associated with worse outcomes than ischemic stroke. However, the unanswered question of long-term DRT surveillance and management is especially important in this population, given that the current strategy is to treat with OAC.

## SUMMARY

Available evidence supports the current recommendation to consider LAAC in patients with AF who have limited options for stroke prevention due to OAC-ineligibility. It is probable that percutaneous LAAC is better than no treatment, and offers a feasible option for stroke prevention in such patients. Ischemic stroke reduction by LAAC in warfarin-eligible patients is inferior to warfarin, although bleeding is reduced. Current data lag behind the rapid evolution of LAAC device design, improvements in implant technique, and changes in standard of care for OAC. Reduced procedural complication and demonstration of at least noninferiority when compared to DOAC treatment are a significant possibility in the near future and these results would rapidly expand the indication to the wider population with AF.

## CLINICS CARE POINTS

- First line stroke prevention in patients with atrial fibrillation should be oral anticoagulation with a DOAC or warfarin.
- LAAC should be considered for patients who are unable to tolerate oral anticoagulation.
- Patients being considered for LAAC should be referred to an experienced, high volume centre as this has been demonstrated to reduce procedural complications.

## DISCLOSURE

K. Saraf has received research funding from Boston Scientific. G.M. Morris has received research funding and honoraria from Boston Scientific and Medtronic, honoraria from Biosense Webster.

## REFERENCES

1. Singer D, Hughes R, Gress D, et al. Stroke Prevention in Atrial Fibrillation Study. Final results. Circulation 1991;84(2):527–39.
2. Connolly SJ, Ezekowitz MD, Yusuf S, et al. Dabigatran versus warfarin in patients with atrial fibrillation. N Engl J Med 2009;361(12):1139–51.
3. Giugliano RP, Ruff CT, Braunwald E, et al. Edoxaban versus warfarin in patients with atrial fibrillation. N Engl J Med 2013;369(22):2093–104.
4. Granger CB, Alexander JH, McMurray JJ, et al. Apixaban versus warfarin in patients with atrial fibrillation. N Engl J Med 2011;365(11):981–92.
5. Patel MR, Mahaffey KW, Garg J, et al. Rivaroxaban versus warfarin in nonvalvular atrial fibrillation. N Engl J Med 2011;365(10):883–91.
6. Saraf K, Morris PD, Garg P, et al. Non-vitamin K antagonist oral anticoagulants (NOACs): clinical evidence and therapeutic considerations. Postgrad Med J 2014;90(1067):520–8.
7. Abushouk AI, Ali AA, Mohamed AA, et al. Rhythm versus rate control for atrial fibrillation: a meta-analysis of randomized controlled trials. Biomed Pharmacol J 2018;11(2):609–20.
8. Thambidorai SK, Murray RD, Parakh K, et al. Utility of transesophageal echocardiography in identification of thrombogenic milieu in patients with atrial fibrillation (an ACUTE ancillary study). Am J Cardiol 2005;96(7):935–41.
9. Stoddard MF, Dawkins PR, Prince CR, et al. Left atrial appendage thrombus is not uncommon in patients with acute atrial fibrillation and a recent embolic event: a transesophageal echocardiographics study. J Am Coll Cardiol 1995;25(2):452–9.
10. Hindricks G, Potpara T, Dagres N, et al. 2020 ESC Guidelines for the diagnosis and management of atrial fibrillation developed in collaboration with the European Association for Cardio-Thoracic Surgery (EACTS). Eur Heart J 2021;42(5):373–498.
11. January CT, Wann LS, Calkins H, et al. 2019 AHA/ACC/HRS focused update of the 2014 AHA/ACC/HRS guideline for the management of patients with atrial fibrillation: A Report of the American College of Cardiology/American Heart Association Task Force on Clinical Practice Guidelines and the Heart Rhythm Society. Heart Rhythm 2019;16(8):e66–93.
12. Ibrahim AM, Tandan N, Koester C, et al. Meta-analysis evaluating outcomes of surgical left atrial appendage occlusion during cardiac surgery. Am J Cardiol 2019;124(8):1218–25.
13. Hanke T. Surgical management of the left atrial appendage: a must or a myth? Eur J Cardiothorac Surg 2018;53(Suppl_1):i33–8.
14. Healey JS, Crystal E, Lamy A, et al. Left Atrial Appendage Occlusion Study (LAAOS): results of a

randomized controlled pilot study of left atrial appendage occlusion during coronary bypass surgery in patients at risk for stroke. Am Heart J 2005;150(2):288–93.

15. Whitlock RP, Belley-Cote EP, Paparella D, et al. Left atrial appendage occlusion during cardiac surgery to prevent stroke. N Engl J Med 2021;384(22):2081–91.

16. Holmes DR Jr, Kar S, Price MJ, et al. Prospective randomized evaluation of the watchman left atrial appendage closure device in patients with atrial fibrillation versus long-term warfarin therapy: the PREVAIL trial. J Am Coll Cardiol 2014;64(1):1–12.

17. Reddy VY, Sievert H, Halperin J, et al. Percutaneous left atrial appendage closure vs warfarin for atrial fibrillation: a randomized clinical trial. JAMA 2014;312(19):1988–98.

18. Osmancik P, Herman D, Neuzil P, et al. Left atrial appendage closure versus direct oral anticoagulants in high-risk patients with atrial fibrillation. J Am Coll Cardiol 2020;75(25):3122–35.

19. Waksman R, Pendyala LK. Overview of the Food and Drug Administration circulatory system devices panel meetings on WATCHMAN left atrial appendage closure therapy. Am J Cardiol 2015;115(3):378–84.

20. Reddy VY, Doshi SK, Kar S, et al. 5-year outcomes after left atrial appendage closure: From the PREVAIL and PROTECT AF Trials. J Am Coll Cardiol 2017;70(24):2964–75.

21. Reddy VY. Medscape. In Defense of Left Atrial Appendage Closure Medscape.com. 2016. Available at: https://www.medscape.com/viewarticle/872433. Accessed November 10, 2021.

22. Jang SJ, Wong SC, Mosadegh B. Leaks after left atrial appendage closure: ignored or neglected? Cardiology 2021;1–8.

23. Huisman MV, Rothman KJ, Paquette M, et al. The changing landscape for stroke prevention in AF: findings From the GLORIA-AF Registry Phase 2. J Am Coll Cardiol 2017;69(7):777–85.

24. Aberegg SK, Hersh AM, Samore MH. Empirical consequences of current recommendations for the design and interpretation of noninferiority trials. J Gen Intern Med 2018;33(1):88–96.

25. Baman JR, Mansour M, Heist EK, et al. Percutaneous left atrial appendage occlusion in the prevention of stroke in atrial fibrillation: a systematic review. Heart Fail Rev 2018;23(2):191–208.

26. Freeman JV, Varosy P, Price MJ, et al. The NCDR left atrial appendage occlusion registry. J Am Coll Cardiol 2020;75(13):1503–18.

27. Kar S, Doshi SK, Sadhu A, et al. Primary outcome evaluation of a next generation left atrial appendage closure device: results from the PINNACLE FLX Trial. Circulation 2021;143(18):1754–62.

28. Srivastava MC, See VY, Dawood MY, et al. A review of the LARIAT device: insights from the cumulative clinical experience. Springerplus 2015;4:522.

29. Nazir S, Ahuja KR, Kolte D, et al. Association of hospital procedural volume with outcomes of percutaneous left atrial appendage occlusion 2021;14(5):554–61.

30. Gupta A, Perera T, Ganesan A, et al. Complications of catheter ablation of atrial fibrillation: a systematic review. Circ Arrhythm Electrophysiol 2013;6(6):1082–8.

31. Wagner G, Steiner S, Gartlehner G, et al. Comparison of transcatheter aortic valve implantation with other approaches to treat aortic valve stenosis: a systematic review and meta-analysis. Syst Rev 2019;8(1):44.

32. Carrion-Camacho MR, Marin-Leon I, Molina-Donoro JM, et al. Safety of permanent pacemaker implantation: a Prospective Study. J Clin Med 2019;8(1):35.

33. Udo E, Hemel Van NM, Zuithoff NPA, et al. Survival and determinants of survival in bradycardia pacemaker recipients: a nationwide cohort study. Eur Heart J 2013;34(Suppl 1):2617.

34. Asad ZUA, Yousif A, Khan MS, et al. Catheter ablation versus medical therapy for atrial fibrillation: a systematic review and meta-analysis of randomized controlled trials. Circ Arrhythm Electrophysiol 2019;12(9):e007414.

35. Mandrola J. Medscape. LAAO vs DOAC: PRAGUE-17 Falls Short: 2020. Available at: www.medscape.com/viewarticle/933641.

36. Boersma LV, Ince H, Kische S, et al. Evaluating real-world clinical outcomes in atrial fibrillation patients receiving the WATCHMAN left atrial appendage closure technology: final 2-year outcome data of the EWOLUTION trial focusing on history of stroke and hemorrhage. Circ Arrhythm Electrophysiol 2019;12(4):e006841.

37. Sedaghat A, Nickenig G, Schrickel JW, et al. Incidence, predictors and outcomes of device-related thrombus after left atrial appendage closure with the WATCHMAN device-Insights from the EWOLUTION real world registry. Catheter Cardiovasc Interv 2021;97(7):E1019–24.

38. Sondergaard L, Wong YH, Reddy VY, et al. Propensity-matched comparison of oral anticoagulation versus antiplatelet therapy after left atrial appendage closure With WATCHMAN. JACC Cardiovasc Interv 2019;12(11):1055–63.

39. Labori F, Bonander C, Persson J, et al. Clinical follow-up of left atrial appendage occlusion in patients with atrial fibrillation ineligible of oral anticoagulation treatment-a systematic review and meta-analysis. J Interv Card Electrophysiol 2021;61(2):215–25.

40. Busu T, Khan SU, Alhajji M, et al. Observed versus expected ischemic and bleeding events following

left atrial appendage occlusion. Am J Cardiol 2020;
125(11):1644–50.

41. Xu H, Xie X, Wang B, et al. Efficacy and safety of
percutaneous left atrial appendage occlusion for
stroke prevention in nonvalvular atrial fibrillation:
a meta-analysis of contemporary studies. Heart
Lung Circ 2016;25(11):1107–17.

42. Ajmal M, Sipra Q, Pecci C, et al. Feasibility of left
atrial appendage closure in atrial fibrillation patients with a history of intracranial bleeding: a systematic review of observational studies. J Interv
Cardiol 2020;2020:1575839.

43. Glikson M, Wolff R, Hindricks G, et al. EHRA/EAPCI
expert consensus statement on catheter-based left
atrial appendage occlusion - an update. EP Europace 2020;22(2):184.

44. Alkhouli M, Busu T, Shah K, et al. Incidence and clinical
impact of device-related thrombus following percutaneous left atrial appendage occlusion: a meta-analysis. JACC Clin Electrophysiol 2018;4(12):1629–37.

45. Dukkipati SR, Kar S, Holmes DR, et al. Device-
related thrombus after left atrial appendage
closure: incidence, predictors, and outcomes. Circulation 2018;138(9):874–85.

# The Strengths and Weaknesses of the LAA Covering Disc Occluders— Conceptually and in Practice

Ivan Wong, MD[a], Apostolos Tzikas, MD, PhD[b],
Lars Søndergaard, MD, DMSc[a],
Ole De Backer, MD, PhD, FESC[a,*]

## KEYWORDS

- Atrial fibrillation • Cardioembolic stroke • Non-pharmacological treatment
- Oral anticoagulant therapy

## KEY POINTS

- Left atrial appendage (LAA) occluders with covering disc design represent a group of established and novel devices.
- LAA occluders with covering disc design have potential advantages in certain complex LAA anatomies and challenging clinical scenarios.
- Device-related thrombosis (DRT) following percutaneous LAA occlusion was shown to be associated with an increased risk of stroke. Patients with pulmonary ridge coverage are reported to have a lower incidence of DRT than those with an uncovered pulmonary ridge.
- Pre-procedural cardiac computed tomography (CT) has the advantage of detailed spatial resolution and 3-dimensional LAA assessment to facilitate correct device sizing, assessment of the surrounding structures, and computational modeling.

## INTRODUCTION

Percutaneous left atrial appendage occlusion (LAAO) is being increasingly recognized as a feasible nonpharmacologic treatment alternative to prevent cardioembolic stroke in patients with nonvalvular atrial fibrillation (NVAF) and contraindications to oral anticoagulant therapy. LAAO has been shown to be noninferior to vitamin K antagonists for stroke prevention in NVAF patients.[1] In the recently published multicenter, randomized, noninferiority PRAGUE-17 trial,[2] a high-risk patient cohort (CHA2DS2-VASc: 4.7 ± 1.5) was randomized to receive LAAO (Amulet, Watchman, or Watchman-FLX

in 61.3%, 35.9%, or 2.8%, respectively) or direct oral anticoagulants (DOACs). LAAO was shown to be noninferior to DOAC treatment in preventing major AF-related cardiovascular, neurologic, and bleeding events. Focusing on endocardial left atrial appendage (LAA) occluders with a covering disc, in a propensity score–matched control cohort, patients with AF who had successful LAAO with the Amplatzer Amulet device (n = 1078) were compared with AF patients (n = 1184) treated by DOACs. The risk of ischemic stroke was comparable between both groups, whereas the risk of major bleeding and all-cause mortality were significantly lower in the LAAO patients.[3]

[a] The Heart Centre, Rigshospitalet, Copenhagen University Hospital, Blegdamsvej 9, Copenhagen 2100, Denmark;
[b] European Interbalkan Medical Centre & AHEPA University Hospital, Asklipiou 10, Thessaloniki 57001, Greece
* Corresponding author. The Heart Centre, Rigshospitalet, University of Copenhagen, Blegdamsvej 9, Copenhagen 2100, Denmark.
E-mail address: ole.debacker@gmail.com

Intervent Cardiol Clin 11 (2022) 185–194
https://doi.org/10.1016/j.iccl.2021.11.010
2211-7458/22/© 2021 Elsevier Inc. All rights reserved.

Endocardial LAA occluders with covering disc encompass a wide range of devices that share the common feature of a distal anchoring "body" and proximal covering "disc" design (Table 1). This is in contrast to the endocardial LAA occluder counterparts with primarily a single "plug" design. In one recent meta-analysis comparing the Amplatzer and Watchman LAAO devices,[4] efficacy and safety were similar between both devices, except for a higher percentage of peridevice leakage (PDL) in the Watchman group.

The current review article aims at providing a comprehensive overview on different aspects of LAA occluders with a covering disc, including (1) device-specific design features, (2) preprocedural imaging updates, (3) intraprocedural technical considerations, and (4) postprocedural follow-up issues.

## LAA OCCLUDERS WITH COVERING DISC DESIGN

### Amplatzer Amulet LAA Occluder

The Amplatzer Amulet LAA occluder (Abbott, MN, USA) is the second-generation Amplatzer LAA occluder, which has replaced the Amplatzer Cardiac Plug (ACP). It is a self-expanding device made of a braided nitinol mesh with 2 polyester patches sewn onto a distal lobe and a proximal disc connected by a short waist (Fig. 1A). The flexible nitinol braid allows the device to conform to different types of LAA anatomy and the device anchors in "landing zones" from 11 to 31 mm in diameter. The minimum required LAA depth is 10 to 12 mm. A proximal Amulet positioning allows device implantation regardless of distal anatomy or existence of multiple lobes. The device adopts an "anchor and seal" approach, with the lobe anchoring in the proximal part of the LAA and the disc sealing the LAA ostium.[5,6]

A Steerable Amplatzer Delivery sheath (14F, Abbott, MN, USA) was recently developed and brought to market. Experience with this steerable delivery sheath is still limited. However, it is expected that use of this steerable sheath may make it easier to obtain coaxial alignment of the LAA closure device and the LAA central axis—this may mitigate the risk of peridevice leaks. In addition, it may simplify complex procedures (eg, in case of a reverse chicken-wing LAA; Fig. 2) and help to correct for suboptimal transseptal puncture.

The Amplatzer Amulet device is one of the most studied LAA occluders on the market. In the Amulet Observational Study,[7] a total of 1088 patients with high risk of stroke and bleeding were enrolled. The implant success rate was 99%, periprocedural complications were 4%, and device-related thrombosis (DRT) rate was 1.6%. At 2 years of follow-up, there was a low ischemic stroke rate of 2.2% per year. Notably, only 11% of patients were discharged on OAC. Nearly 60% of patients were on single antiplatelet agent or no antithrombotic medication at 1 to 3 months after LAAO, and this proportion increased to 84% at 2 years.

Recently, the results of the Amulet IDE trial were presented at the ESC congress 2021 and simultaneously published in Circulation.[8] This large randomized controlled trial including 1878 patients was designed to evaluate the safety and effectiveness of the dual-seal mechanism of the Amulet LAA occluder compared with the Watchman device (2.5 generation, Boston Scientific, USA). The Amulet LAA occluder was shown to be noninferior for safety and effectiveness of stroke prevention compared with the Watchman device, and superior for LAA closure (mechanism of action). Peridevice leaks $\geq$ 3 mm at 45 days post-LAA closure were seen in 25% of patients in the Watchman cohort versus only in 10% of patients in the Amulet cohort ($P<.0001$). Complete LAA closure without any residual jets was observed in 46% and 63% of patients in the Watchman and Amulet cohorts, respectively. Based on these outcomes, the Amulet LAA occluder obtained FDA approval in the United States.

Another important randomized controlled trial investigating the Amulet device, in which patients are currently actively enrolled, is the CATALYST trial (NCT04226547). This global multicenter CATALYST trial will compare the effectiveness of the Amplatzer Amulet device to DOACs as an alternative treatment option in an expanded population of atrial fibrillation patients with CHADS-VASc $\geq$ 3 and eligible for long-term DOAC therapy.

### LAmbre LAA Occluder

The LAmbre LAA closure system (LifeTech Scientific Co., Ltd., China) is a self-expanding, nitinol-based meshwork that consists of a hook-embedded umbrella connected to a fabric cover through a short central waist (Fig. 1B). The LAmbre device is available in 15 diameter sizes with reference to the umbrella part (16–36 mm). The device has 2 configurations: a "standard" one targeting single-lobe LAAs and a "special" one targeting multilobe LAA anatomies. There are 8 stabilizing double-hook systems with big hooks (or folded barbs) catching the pectinate muscles in the LAA, whereas the small shoulder

**Table 1**
**Left atrial appendage occluders with covering disc design**

|  | Manufacturer | Design | Size (mm) | Sheath (F) |
| --- | --- | --- | --- | --- |
| Amplatzer Amulet | Abbott | Lobe and disc | 16, 18, 20, 22, 25, 28, 31, 34 | 12–14 |
| LAmbre | Lifetech Scientific | Umbrella and cover | 16, 18, 20, 22, 24, 26, 28, 30, 32, 34, 36 | 8–10 |
| OMEGA | Eclipse Medical | Cup and disc | 14, 16, 18, 20, 22, 24, 26, 28, 30 | 14 |
| SeaLA | Hangzhou Valued Medtech | Double disc | 16, 18, 20, 22, 24, 26, 28, 30, 32, 34, 36 | 9–12 |

hooks engage into the LAA wall to mitigate the risk of device migration/embolization.[5,9] During the procedure, the delivery sheath is fixated at the very proximal portion of the LAA, and the umbrella is deployed at the landing zone by pushing forward the delivery cable. The fabric cover is then released by unsheathing to cover the LAA ostium. The device is fully recapturable and repositionable.

In a prospective, multicenter clinical study,[10] the LAA was successfully occluded by the LAmbre device in 152 patients (99.4%). Serious complications occurred in 5 patients (3.3%). During the 12-month follow-up, ischemic stroke occurred in 2 patients, 1 patient had incomplete LAA sealing (residual flow >3 mm), and there was no device embolization. The device obtained CE mark approval in 2016.

### OMEGA LAA Occluder

The OMEGA LAAO device (Eclipse Medical, Ireland) is a novel self-expanding platinum-coated nitinol "disc-and-cup" occluder (Fig. 1C). Unique features of the device are: (1) a double-layered and "self-retaining" inverted cup with 6–10 circumferentially interspersed hooks, which promotes device stability into the neck of the LAA; (2) a very flexible "waist," which allows the device to conform to the most complex LAA morphologies; and (3) a platinum coating, which should provide favorable biocompatibility. Nine device sizes ranging from 14 to 30 mm (in 2 mm increments) are available and referred to by the maximal diameter of the cup, allowing anchoring in LAAs with a landing zone diameter between 10.5 and 25.5 mm. A minimum LAA depth of 10 mm to 15 mm is required for the OMEGA 14 to 22 mm devices and 24 to 30 mm devices, respectively.

Based on in vitro bench tests with the OMEGA device in human 3-dimensional LAA models with different LAA morphologies,[11] it could be determined that selection of the OMEGA device size should be best based on the maximum LAA ostium diameter and the LAA landing zone as measured at a depth of 10 to 15 mm from the LAA ostium. A device compression rate and, hence, landing zone over-sizing of 10% to 25% resulted in proper device anchoring.

In the first-in-human clinical trial,[12] the primary efficacy endpoint of LAAO at 30 to 90 days was obtained in all recipients with complete LAA closure in 11 patients (85%) and a small residual PDL less than 3 mm in 2 patients (15%). The primary safety endpoint was noted in 1 patient who developed a mild pericardial effusion, which was initially managed conservatively but drained percutaneously 6 weeks later.

The OMEGA device obtained CE mark approval in 2020 and is currently further investigated in a European multicenter postmarket clinical follow-up study.

### SeaLA LAA Occluder

The SeaLA LAA occluder (Hangzhou Valued Medtech Co., Ltd.) is a self-expanding, nitinol-based device, which consists of 2 parts: a distal anchoring part and a more proximal "plate" to obtain sealing (Fig. 1D).[5] The nitinol braiding mesh for both components helps to adapt to different LAA morphologies. The device also adopts the "anchor and seal" principle. The distal part has 9 hooks to assure anchoring and the proximal plate has a small, tapered waist that potentially optimizes LAA wall apposition and, hence, should provide better sealing. The device is fully retrievable and repositionable. As the device does not need a deep LAA implantation, a proximal implant position allows for placement regardless of distal anatomy or lobe morphology. Initial experience with 11 human implants between 2016 and 2017 in Argentina and China were all successful. No complications or residual leaks were reported.

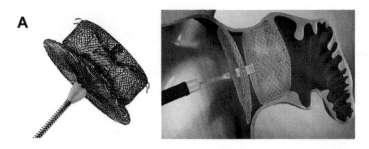

**A**

Fig. 1. LAA occluders with covering disc design. (A) Amplatzer Amulet LAA occluder. (B) LAmbre LAA occluder. (C) OMEGA LAA occluder. (D) SeaLA LAA occluder. SRIC, self-retaining inverted cup.

**B**

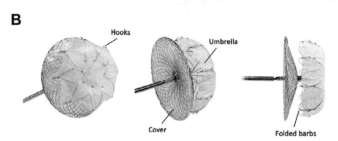

Hooks

Umbrella

Cover

Folded barbs

**C**

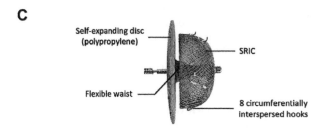

Self-expanding disc (polypropylene)

SRIC

Flexible waist

8 circumferentially interspersed hooks

**D**

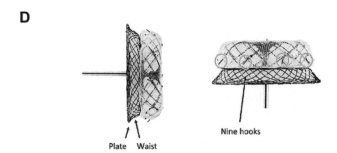

Nine hooks

Plate   Waist

## PREPROCEDURAL IMAGING UPDATES

The LAA has a complex and highly heterogenous anatomy. Accurate sizing of the LAA is therefore essential when performing percutaneous LAAO. Traditionally, 2-dimensional transesophageal echocardiography (TEE) has been the officially recommended imaging modality in LAAO preprocedural planning. However, other imaging modalities could also be used. In addition, complex LAA morphology requires more detailed spatial resolution and 3-dimensional assessments to reduce the risk of incorrect sizing. As reported in an LAA imaging study, only 33 of 58 LAA sizings (57%) by TEE would have led to a correct selection of the LAA closure device size, whereas in the case of cardiac computed tomography (CT)-based sizing, 48 of 58 LAA sizings (83%) would have resulted in a correct device size selection.[13] Another randomized trial highlighted that cardiac CT improved preprocedural LAAO device size selection accuracy compared with 2-dimensional TEE, resulting in shorter procedure times.[14]

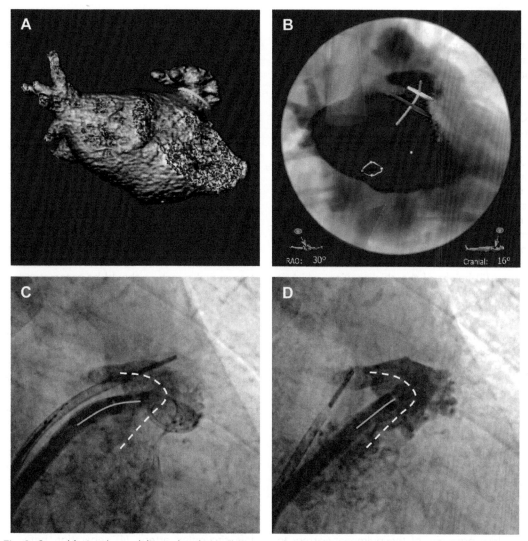

**Fig. 2.** Steerable Amplatzer delivery sheath. (*A, B*) Preprocedural cardiac computed tomography imaging showing a reverse chicken-wing LAA and the optimal implantation view in which the LAA ostium and landing zone could be aligned (RAO 30°, cranial 16°). (*C, D*) Coaxial alignment of the LAA central axis and delivery sheath could be obtained following extension of the Amplatzer Steerable Delivery Sheath.

Both LAA ostium and landing zone measurements are typically required for device size selection of LAA occluders with covering disc design. The position and definition of the landing zone are different for each of the aforementioned LAA occluders, but the methodological approach to define the landing zone is similar.[15] Of note, studies have shown that there are differences in measurements obtained with different imaging modalities, with cardiac CT giving the largest measurements, followed by 3-dimensional TEE, and then 2-dimensional TEE and angiography.[16] Cardiac CT-based perimeter-derived mean diameter has been shown to be the best parameter to guide device

size selection for "closed-end" devices (eg, Amulet).[13] In fact, for 2-dimensional imaging modalities, LAA diameters tend to be underestimated, and LAA largest diameters, therefore, seem to be the best option for device sizing. For cardiac CT-based sizing recommendations, data are currently more robust for the Amulet device. As mentioned, the perimeter-derived mean LAA diameter derived from cardiac CT has been shown to be the best parameter for device size selection and LAA sealing. An updated sizing chart for the Amulet device was recently published.[16] Using the cardiac CT LAA mean diameter, an upsize by 2 to 5 mm for Amulet device size selection would be appropriate, as long as this device is not smaller than the largest LAA diameter at the landing zone. Importantly, operators are recommended not to choose a device smaller than the maximal LAA diameter at the landing zone.

Certain specific LAA anatomies warrant separate consideration in imaging assessment. Chicken-wing LAAs are defined by an early (<20 mm from the ostium) and severe bend (>90°) of the main lobe. Cardiac CT with 3-dimensional postprocessing analysis typically allows better visual assessment of this complex morphology. Device sizing is different from the conventional approach. Four main measurements have been suggested: (1) the maximum internal lobe diameter measured at the bending of the LAA lobe ("the chicken-wing ridge")—the device lobe should be at least 20% to 30% larger; (2) height of the chicken-wing, which is less important as long as the device lobe is considerably larger than the ridge maximal diameter; (3) width of the chicken-wing since the distal body of the device needs to fit inside the chicken-wing; and (4) maximal diameter of LAA ostium as the size of the device should be chosen in such way that the proximal covering disc can cover the LAA ostium.[17]

Preprocedural cardiac CT has an additional advantage as it gives the opportunity to make a detailed assessment of the surrounding structures adjacent to the LAA. In particular, it is recommended to actively screen for close proximity between the pulmonary artery and the anticipated LAA occluder landing zone on preprocedural imaging. "Cuddling lobe orientation" of the Amulet device with the pulmonary artery (ie, close proximity of the pulmonary artery to the Amulet lobe in both its middle and distal part) has been described to be associated with device-related pulmonary artery injury and late pericardial effusion.[18] Alternative LAA occluders with different landing zone depth requirements or with a different anchoring mechanism may therefore be considered in this particular setting.

Cardiac CT is also increasingly recognized as a valuable tool in LAA imaging assessment. Recently, a cardiac CT-based computational model (FEops HEARTguide, Belgium) has been developed to simulate the deployment of the 2 most commonly used LAA occluders into patient-specific LAA anatomies. Computational models can provide operators additional insights into patient-specific anatomy and its interaction with the implanted device. It was shown that patient-specific computational modeling allows accurate prediction of LAAO device deformation and apposition.[19] Computational modeling may therefore potentiate more accurate LAAO device size selection and better preprocedural planning.

## INTRAPROCEDURAL TECHNICAL CONSIDERATIONS

First of all, an optimal transseptal puncture to achieve delivery sheath coaxiality with the LAA central axis is important as this facilitates device implantation and increases the chances of obtaining complete LAA closure. In most LAAO cases, an inferoposterior transseptal puncture should be aimed for. However, in some specific cases such as reverse chicken-wing LAAs or LAAs in which the proximal part makes a posterior bend, a more central-inferior transseptal puncture should be recommended. This again highlights the advantage of preprocedural cardiac CT assessment, which can accurately predict the optimal transseptal puncture site in relation to the trajectory of the LAA neck and ostium.

The conventional steps of device deployment vary according to the LAA occluder used and each manufacturer has unique implantation criteria for optimal deployment before release of the device. However, the 5 signs of a good implantation and stability for the Amulet device are also applicable to the other covering disc LAA occluders: (1) sufficient compression of the distal anchoring lobe or "body"; (2) axis of the distal anchoring lobe or "body" in line with the axis of the LAA neck; (3) two-third of the distal anchoring lobe or "body" distal to the left circumflex artery; (4) separation between the distal anchoring lobe or "body" and the disc; and (5) slight concavity of the device disc, thereby restoring the concavity of the left atrial (LA) wall. A tug-test is often also performed to confirm good anchoring and stability of the LAA occluder, before final release from the delivery cable.

LAA occluders with a covering disc design may have potential advantages in more complex LAA anatomies. For instance, a chicken-wing LAA anatomy as mentioned earlier may require a different implantation technique. The "sandwich technique" is indicated in case the neck (landing zone) of the chicken-wing LAA is shallow (<15–20 mm). Its main characteristic is that the device lobe is not implanted in the standard LAA neck position but the lobe rather lies along the length of the LAA body (wing), resulting in "sandwiching" the proximal part of LAA between the device lobe and disc (Fig. 3).[6]

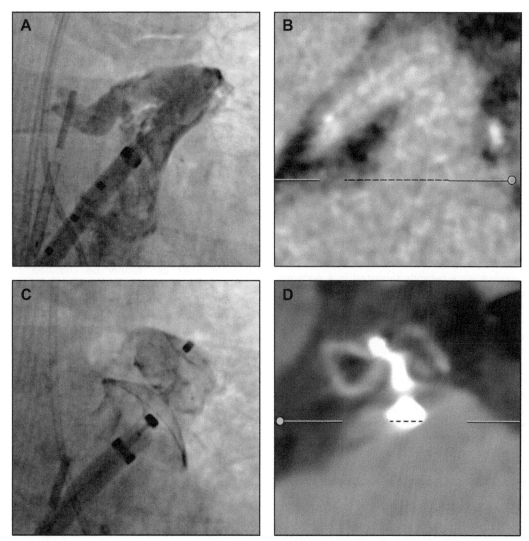

Fig. 3. Case example of the "sandwich" implantation technique using an Amplatzer Amulet LAA occluder in a reversed chicken-wing LAA anatomy. (A) Angiogram showing a reverse chicken-wing LAA anatomy. (B) Corresponding CT reconstruction of the reverse chicken-wing LAA anatomy. (C) "Sandwich" implantation technique using the Amplatzer Amulet device. (D) Postprocedural cardiac CT reconstruction showing complete LAA sealing without contrast leakage.

Since this particular implantation technique and the final device position are substantially different from the standard technique, the typical signs of stability (device compression in particular) may not be present in some cases. One important aspect is to ensure there is good wall apposition of the device lobe at the base of the wing. A stability test with gentle backward tension of the delivery cable is also generally recommended to ensure device stability. It is also crucial to confirm that no part of the device lobe is protruding into the LA creating a potential risk for device embolization. Freixa and colleagues[17] recently reported the procedural and follow-up outcome of 190 patients undergoing percutaneous LAAO using the "sandwich technique." Procedures were all done with LAA occluders with covering disc design (Amulet device in 85% and ACP in 15%). Clinical outcomes at follow-up showed similar mortality, stroke, and bleeding rates compared with previous conventional LAAO series; and the incidence of DRT and PDL at follow-up was 2.8% and 1.2%, respectively. Notably, the "sandwich technique" can theoretically be performed with any LAA occluder that has a "disc" and "lobe," but not with a single "plug" configuration LAA occluder.

Percutaneous LAA closure in patients with LAA thrombus represents another challenging scenario in which covering disc LAA occluders may have potential advantages. Persistent LAA thrombus has traditionally been a contraindication to LAAO because of concern about systemic embolization. These patients have also been excluded from major LAAO trials. LAAO in this high-risk cohort requires extra caution and modification of the standard implantation technique. LAA angiography and guidewire or catheter manipulation inside the LAA should be kept to a minimum. Careful advancement of the delivery sheath inside the LA followed by cautious advancement of the partially open "ball configuration" of the device toward the LAA is recommended. Feasibility and safety of LAAO procedures in patients with persistent LAA thrombus were recently reported in a systemic review.[20] LAA occluders with covering disc (Amulet, ACP, and LAmbre) were used in 85% of cases. Most patients had a distally located thrombus in the LAA. LAAO devices were implanted in all cases without any procedural complications. A cerebral protection device was used in 29% of patients. One stroke (1.7%) and 2 DRT (3.4%) were noted during the mean follow-up of 3.4 ± 7 months. LAA occluders with a covering disc design and a short length of the distal anchoring lobe or "body" allow for a shallow deployment at the most proximal part of the LAA without having to engage the distal LAA, and potentially avoid any contact with the LAA thrombus. Nevertheless, proximal LAA thrombus at the landing zone remains a contraindication to LAAO, and the presence of LA, mitral valve, or left ventricular thrombus should always be excluded before LAAO.[21]

Finally, the use of intracardiac echocardiography (ICE) for LAAO intraprocedural imaging guidance has become routine in many centers. The capacity to avoid general anesthesia, TEE, and provide echocardiographic guidance during the procedure are the main advantages of ICE. Studies have shown comparable procedural outcomes with TEE or ICE guidance for LAAO with LAA occluders with covering disc design. In the Amulet Observational Study, LAAO procedures guided by ICE and TEE resulted in comparable clinical event rates and LAA closure rates, without differences in procedural or vascular complications.[22] All institutions that use ICE guidance for LAAO rely on preprocedural cardiac CT or 3-dimensional TEE for device sizing and LAA morphology assessment, because sizing and characterization of complex LAA anatomies are limited by single-plane and 2-dimensional images of ICE.

## POSTPROCEDURAL FOLLOW-UP
### Device-Related Thrombosis

DRT is a potential complication during follow-up after LAAO. The incidence of DRT is generally reported between 2% and 5% in the literature.[23] Most patients with DRT are diagnosed during early routine follow-up imaging. Either follow-up TEE or cardiac CT can be used to identify DRT. DRT on TEE is defined as a homogenous echo-dense mass visible in different planes with independent motion and adherence to the atrial surface of the LAAO occluder. DRT on cardiac CT is defined as hypoattenuated thickening (HAT) on the atrial surface of the LAAO occluder. HAT can further be classified into high-grade or low-grade DRT according to morphology and thickness.[24]

In the Amulet Observational Study,[23] 18% of DRT patients had an ischemic stroke, all within 3 months of DRT diagnosis. Patients with a DRT were at a greater risk for ischemic stroke or transient ischemic attack compared with non-DRT patients in the study. Notably, the left upper pulmonary vein ridge was not covered by the Amulet disc in 82% of DRT patients, indicating suboptimal device implantation, with most thrombus developing in the untrabeculated triangular area of the LAA ostium between the pulmonary vein ridge and the superior edge of the disc of the LAA occluder.

Subsequently, Freixa and colleagues[25] evaluated the impact of left upper pulmonary ridge coverage on both clinical and imaging follow-up outcomes in patients undergoing LAAO. All LAAO procedures were conducted with LAA occluders with covering disc design (ACP in 10%, Amulet in 75%, and LAmbre in 15%). Patients with a covered pulmonary ridge presented a lower incidence of DRT (1%) than those with an uncovered pulmonary ridge (27%) (P<.001). Most DRTs were located in the triangular area at the pulmonary ridge. In addition, a history of previous ischemic stroke and the presence of spontaneous echo contrast were also identified as independent risk factors for DRT.

From a procedural point of view, coverage of the pulmonary ridge with the disc should always be aimed for with LAA occluders with a covering disc, except in cases where there is prominent pulmonary ridge protrusion or a huge LAA ostium beyond the maximal size of the covering disc. Optimal (preprocedural) device size selection and refinements in LAAO implantation technique may improve LAA sealing, potentially reducing the risk of DRT formation.

### Peridevice Leak

Incomplete LAA closure or persistent leaks around the LAA occluder are not uncommon. PDL mostly is associated with device malposition, device compression <10%, larger LAA dimensions, or complex LAA anatomies.[26] However, so far, no single study has reported an association between PDL size on TEE and clinical outcomes after LAAO.[27]

PDL can either be detected by TEE or cardiac CT.[28] In a recently published comparative imaging study in LAAO patients performed with the ACP/Amulet device,[26] there were substantial discrepancies in detection and quantification of PDL by TEE versus cardiac CT, with a markedly higher incidence of PDL detected by cardiac CT. Nevertheless, the presence of a severe PDL by cardiac CT or TEE was not associated with worse 4-year clinical outcomes. Based on available evidence in the literature, it is reasonable to remain conservative for PDL of less than 5 mm following LAAO with any type of LAA occluder. For PDL of ≥5 mm, management with oral anticoagulation would be reasonable (unless there is a high bleeding risk), whereas percutaneous PDL closure may be considered on an individualized basis.[27]

### SUMMARY

LAA occluders with covering disc design represent a group of established and novel devices. Undoubtedly, this category of devices has certain advantages in complex LAA anatomy and some challenging clinical scenarios. On the other hand, deployment techniques may be less straightforward as compared with a single "plug" design device. Data are emerging on the clinical safety and efficacy of some novel devices in this category.

### DISCLOSURE

Dr. Tzikas, Søndergaard and De Backer received institutional research grants and consulting fees from Abbott.

### REFERENCES

1. Holmes DR Jr, Doshi SK, Kar S, et al. Left atrial appendage closure as an alternative to warfarin for stroke prevention in atrial fibrillation: a patient-level meta-analysis. J Am Coll Cardiol 2015;65(24):2614–23.
2. Osmancik P, Herman D, Neuzil P, et al. PRAGUE-17 trial investigators. left atrial appendage closure versus direct oral anticoagulants in high-risk patients with atrial fibrillation. J Am Coll Cardiol 2020;75(25):3122–35.
3. Nielsen-Kudsk JE, Korsholm K, Damgaard D, et al. Clinical outcomes associated with left atrial appendage occlusion versus direct oral anticoagulation in atrial fibrillation. JACC Cardiovasc Interv 2021;14(1):69–78.
4. Basu Ray I, Khanra D, Shah S, et al. Meta-analysis comparing watchman and amplatzer devices for stroke prevention in atrial fibrillation. Front Cardiovasc Med 2020;7:89.
5. Chow DHF, Wong YH, Park JW, et al. An overview of current and emerging devices for percutaneous left atrial appendage closure. Trends Cardiovasc Med 2019;29(4):228–36.
6. Tzikas A, Gafoor S, Meerkin D, et al. Left atrial appendage occlusion with the Amplatzer Amulet device: an expert consensus step-by-step approach. EuroIntervention 2016;11(13):1512–21.
7. Hildick-Smith D, Landmesser U, Camm AJ, et al. Left atrial appendage occlusion with the Amplatzer™ Amulet™ device: full results of the prospective global observational study. Eur Heart J 2020;41(30):2894–901.
8. Lakkireddy D, Thaler D, Ellis CR, et al. Amplatzer™ Amulet™ left atrial appendage occluder versus Watchman device™ for stroke prophylaxis (AMULET IDE): a randomized controlled trial. Circulation 2021. https://doi.org/10.1161/CIRCULATIONAHA.121.057063.
9. Cruz-Gonzalez I, Moreno-Samos JC, Rodriguez-Collado J, et al. Percutaneous closure of left atrial appendage with complex anatomy using a LAmbre Device. JACC Cardiovasc Interv 2017;10(4):e37–9.
10. Huang H, Liu Y, Xu Y, et al. Percutaneous left atrial appendage closure with the lambre device for stroke prevention in atrial fibrillation: a prospective, multicenter clinical study. JACC Cardiovasc Interv 2017;10(21):2188–94.
11. De Backer O, Hafiz H, Fabre A, et al. State-of-the-art preclinical testing of the OMEGATM left atrial appendage occluder. Catheter Cardiovasc Interv 2020. https://doi.org/10.1002/ccd.29331.
12. Wilkins B, Srimahachota S, De Backer O, et al. First-in-human results of the OMEGA™ Left Atrial Appendage Occluder for Patients with Non-Valvular Atrial Fibrillation. EuroIntervention 2021;17:e376–9.
13. Chow DH, Bieliauskas G, Sawaya FJ, et al. A comparative study of different imaging modalities for successful percutaneous left atrial appendage closure. Open Heart 2017;4(2):e000627.
14. Eng MH, Wang DD, Greenbaum AB, et al. Prospective, randomized comparison of 3-dimensional computed tomography guidance versus TEE data for left atrial appendage occlusion (PRO3DLAAO). Catheter Cardiovasc Interv 2018;92(2):401–7.

15. Korsholm K, Berti S, Iriart X, et al. Expert recommendations on cardiac computed tomography for planning transcatheter left atrial appendage occlusion. JACC Cardiovasc Interv 2020;13(3):277–92.

16. Freixa X, Aminian A, Tzikas A, et al. Left atrial appendage occlusion with the Amplatzer Amulet: update on device sizing. J Interv Card Electrophysiol 2020;59(1):71–8.

17. Freixa X, Tzikas A, Aminian A, et al. Left atrial appendage occlusion in chicken-wing anatomies: Imaging assessment, procedural, and clinical outcomes of the "sandwich technique. Catheter Cardiovasc Interv 2021. https://doi.org/10.1002/ccd.29546.

18. Pracoń R, De Backer O, Konka M, et al. Imaging risk features for device related pulmonary artery injury after left atrial appendage closure with Amplatzer™ Amulet™ device. Catheter Cardiovasc Interv 2020. https://doi.org/10.1002/ccd.29393.

19. Bavo AM, Wilkins BT, Garot P, et al. Validation of a computational model aiming to optimize preprocedural planning in percutaneous left atrial appendage closure. J Cardiovasc Comput Tomogr 2020;14(2):149–54.

20. Sharma SP, Cheng J, Turagam MK, et al. Feasibility of left atrial appendage occlusion in left atrial appendage thrombus: a systematic review. JACC Clin Electrophysiol 2020;6(4):414–24.

21. Bajoras V, Vejlstrup NG, Wong I, et al. Unusual finding during screening for intracardiac thrombus in patients referred for percutaneous left atrial appendage closure. Kardiol Pol 2021. https://doi.org/10.33963/KP.15958.

22. Nielsen-Kudsk JE, Berti S, De Backer O, et al. Use of intracardiac compared with transesophageal echocardiography for left atrial appendage occlusion in the amulet observational study. JACC Cardiovasc Interv 2019;12(11):1030–9.

23. Aminian A, Schmidt B, Mazzone P, et al. Incidence, characterization, and clinical impact of device-related thrombus following left atrial appendage occlusion in the prospective global AMPLATZER Amulet Observational Study. JACC Cardiovasc Interv 2019;12(11):1003–14.

24. Korsholm K, Jensen JM, Nørgaard BL, et al. Detection of device-related thrombosis following left atrial appendage occlusion: a comparison between cardiac computed tomography and transesophageal echocardiography. Circ Cardiovasc Interv 2019;12(9):e008112.

25. Freixa X, Cepas-Guillen P, Flores-Umanzor E, et al. Pulmonary ridge coverage and device-related thrombosis after left atrial appendage occlusion. EuroIntervention 2021;16(15):e1288–94.

26. Korsholm K, Jensen JM, Nørgaard BL, et al. Peridevice leak following amplatzer left atrial appendage occlusion: cardiac computed tomography classification and clinical outcomes. JACC Cardiovasc Interv 2021;14(1):83–93.

27. Raphael CE, Friedman PA, Saw J, et al. Residual leaks following percutaneous left atrial appendage occlusion: assessment and management implications. EuroIntervention 2017;13(10):1218–25.

28. Tzikas A, Holmes DR Jr, Gafoor S, et al. Percutaneous left atrial appendage occlusion: the Munich consensus document on definitions, endpoints and data collection requirements for clinical studies. EuroIntervention 2016;12(1):103–11.

# Left Atrial Appendage Occlusion Strengths and Weaknesses of the Lobe-Only Occluder Concept in Theory and in Practice

Kolja Sievert, MD[a], Lluis Asmarats, MD, PhD[b],
Dabit Arzamendi, MD, PhD[b,c],*

## KEYWORDS

- Left atrial appendage • Atrial fibrillation • Stroke • LAA occluder • Nondisk LAAO devices

## KEY POINTS

- Differences in the design of left atrial appendage occluders might have an impact on outcomes (DRT, leak, or embolization).
- Devices with no external disk have the advantage of a lower interference with surrounding structures and a smaller surface interacting with blood, which might have an impact on DRT.
- The absence of the disk is a limitation in some scenarios or anatomies and a higher incidence of peridevice leak might be observed.

## INTRODUCTION: RATIONALE FOR THE NONDISK LEFT ATRIAL APPENDAGE OCCLUSION DEVICES

Left atrial appendage (LAA) closure aims to eliminate the stasis component of Virchow triad by eliminating a cul-de-sac that favors thrombosis, particularly when atrial contractility becomes inefficient, such as in atrial fibrillation (AF). Early surgical experience demonstrated that LAA ligation reduced the incidence of stroke in patients operated for concomitant mitral pathology.[1] However, as pulmonary vein ablation extended the use of percutaneous access to the left atrium to treat patients with AF,[2] it was only a matter of time before the first devices to occlude the LAA were developed. The first transcatheter LAA closure was performed with the PLATOO, a single lobe with no-added disk, device. The initial results reported a high success rate, especially considering that it was the first-in-class, encouraging development of the procedure and the device concept.[3]

Subsequently, other appendage closure devices were produced, which mostly included an internal lobe along with an external disk mimicking the classical two-disk Amplatzer devices. This strategy has proven useful to treat septal defects with a surrounding wall that allows the double disk system to anchor. However, in the case of the LAA, where there is no true wall but rather a cul-de-sac, anchoring becomes a challenging issue. For this reason, all appendage closure devices searched for different designs to guarantee adequate anchorage to avoid embolization, and most resorted to the use of additional small hooks.

[a] CardioVascular Center Frankfurt (CVC), St. Catherine Hospital, Seckbacher Landstraße 65, 60389 Frankfurt am Main, Germany; [b] Department of Cardiology, Hospital de la Santa Creu I Sant Pau, Sant Antoni Maria Claret 167, Barcelona 08025, Spain; [c] Centro de Investigación Biomédica en Red de Enfermedades Cardiovasculares (CIBERCV)
* Corresponding author. Department of Cardiology, Hospital de la Santa Creu I Sant Pau, Sant Antoni Maria Claret 167, Barcelona 08025, Spain.
E-mail address: darzamendi@santpau.cat

Intervent Cardiol Clin 11 (2022) 195–203
https://doi.org/10.1016/j.iccl.2021.11.004
2211-7458/22/© 2021 Elsevier Inc. All rights reserved.

This raises the question whether an external disk is needed routinely. Supporters of that approach attest that on many occasions the disk achieves a more complete seal than a simple lobe, by covering the ostium of the appendage and thus reducing peridevice leakage. A dual lobe-disk device strategy is useful in those shallow multilobed appendages, where the lobe is used for anchoring in one of the LAA recesses, and the sealing of the ostium is achieved by the disk. Moreover, the disk can also render coverage of the pulmonary ridge, an aspect that has been associated with a lower risk of device thrombosis.[4]

Conversely, detractors argue that the external disk implies the use of more foreign material permanently in the patient, which could increase the rate of device thrombosis. Most devices lack disk articulation and, in angulated appendages, it may be difficult to perfectly align the disk with the ostium, creating recesses that could favor thrombosis. Finally, and perhaps the main argument for this line of thinking, the disk can potentially interfere with neighboring structures, such as the pulmonary veins or the mitral valve, making the procedure more challenging.

In summary, devices that use the lobe-disk design have the advantage that the internal lobe can simply serve as an anchor and closure is made with the disk, whereas only lobe devices have to achieve anchoring and sealing of the appendage simultaneously. The key in this latter type of device derives from the conformability of the device in the appendage, where an optimal adjustment to the LAA anatomy enables better anchorage and sealing simultaneously. In any case, the ultimate goals of all LAA closure devices are: (1) to achieve an adequate seal (with no residual peridevice leaks), (2) to ensure device stability (to avoid embolization), and (3) to avoid device-related thrombus (DRT) generation. This review provides a detailed overview of the nondisk devices in this regard.

## DEVICE OVERVIEW

There are currently two main transcatheter intracardiac principles for LAA closure: the pacifier principle (lobe-disk design) and the plug principle (single lobe design). The most well studied of each category are the Watchman/Watchman FLX (Boston Scientific Corporation) Occluder (plug principle) and the Amplatzer Amulet (Abbott Vascular) Occluder (pacifier principle). Other LAA occluders designed after the plug principle include the WaveCrest (Biosense Webster, Inc., a Johnson & Johnson company)

Occluder, Occlutech Plus (Occlutech International AB), Prolipsis (Custom Medical Devices), Irisseal, Aurigen (Aurigen Medical Limited), Conformal (Conformal Medical Inc), Flow Medtech (Venturelab), and MemoLefort (Lepu Medical Technology). Other LAA occluders designed after the pacifier principle are the Occlutech Vario, LAmbre (Lifetech Scientific Co., Ltd.), Pfm Medical (Pfm Medical), Ultraseal (Cardia, Inc.), SeaLA (Hangzhou Valued Medtech Co., Ltd), and the Omega (Vascular Innovations Co. Ltd.). The Cormos device belongs in both categories because there are two versions under evaluation. Devices designed for an epicardial approach to LAA closure are Lariat and AEGIS. An intracardiac Occluder with a novel concept is the Append Medical using intracardiac ligation of the LAA. Despite the long list of LAA occlusion (LAAO) devices, many of them are not currently on the market. We focus on those with the plug principle that are still available in the market.

The Watchman FLX LAAO is an example of the plug principle. It is the new generation of the Watchman, which received CE mark in 2005 and Food and Drug Administration approval in 2015. The Watchman FLX received initial CE mark in 2015 but required a redesign because of increased device embolization. After redesign, the Watchman FLX received CE mark in 2019 and Food and Drug Administration approval in 2020 for patients with nonvalvular AF. The Watchman FLX is a nitinol device that is implanted percutaneously to seal the LAA. The device radially expands to maintain position in the LAA. Changed features of the device are an increase in the number of struts from 10 to 18 (in the nitinol frame), which gives the device 80% more contact points against the LAA ostium, enhancing the seal because of a more uniform coverage. There are two rows of J-anchors, which have been designed so that the Watchman FLX is fully retrievable and can be redeployed without damaging the anchors. Two-thirds of the device is covered in fabric (polyethylene terephthalate) to facilitate sealing in case of a proximal shoulder, as a filter to prevent embolization of thrombus from within the LAA, and to facilitate endothelialization. The occluder is shorter in comparison with the previous generation and allows for a shallow deployment by advancing the partially deployed device into the LAA (push forward implantation technique). It is available in five sizes (20, 24, 27, 31, and 35 mm) and is more flexible in regard to sizing overlap facilitating closure of larger and smaller appendages. The threaded insert used to connect the delivery system is embedded inside the device to reduce exposed metal to the left atrium (Fig. 1).

The WaveCrest is another occluder with a plug principle. It is made of a nitinol frame where the left atrial side is covered in expanded polytetra-fluoroethylene (ePTFE) to prevent thrombus formation and the LAA side has a foam layer to accelerate endothelization. The occluder has no pores and is immediately occlusive. It requires a short landing zone (<10 mm) and allows for a proximal implantation technique. The anchoring of the WaveCrest is accomplished by compression and small anchor hooks. The anchor hooks can be deployed independently from the device placement. This occluder only has one short sealing zone requiring exact placement of the device without any malalignment. The device is available in three sizes (22, 27, and 32 mm).

## SPECIFIC FEATURES OF THE OCCLUDER-ONLY CONCEPT

### Implantation Success and Device Embolization

There was a general belief that the pacifier-type devices should allow coverage of a wider range of LAA anatomies, and that this would imply a higher closure success rate. These devices might allow coverage of shallow appendages with short depth, which could not be more challenging for single-lobe devices. Yet this theoretical advantage appears to have only a small clinical impact. The overall implantation success rate of LAA closure is similar between device strategies - the Amulet/Amplatzer Cardiac Plug with a success rate between 95.4%[5] and 99%,[6] whereas the Watchman FLX has a success rate between 96%[7] and 100%.[8] In the head-to-head Amulet IDE study, the implant success rate of

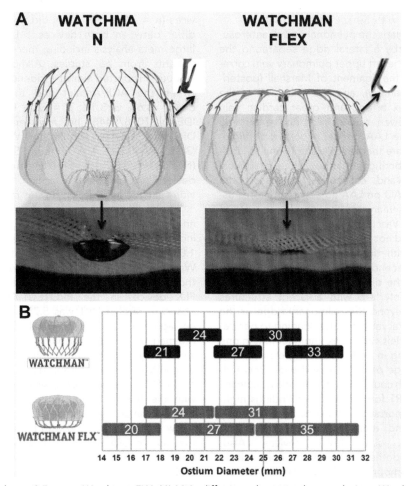

Fig. 1. Watchman 2.5 versus Watchman FLX. (A) Main differences between the two devices: Watchman FLX presents a closed distal end, it is shorter, and has two rows of J-shaped anchors (18 total vs 10 straight in the Watchman 2.5) and a recessed metal screw in the proximal face. (B) Device sizing chart: Watchman FLX offers a wider LAA ostium range (from 14 to 31.5 mm).

the Amulet was 98.4% compared with 96.4% in the Watchman 2.5 group.[9] Stability is the other side of the implantation coin. Embolization rates for the ACP/Amulet range from 0.1%[6] to 3.9%.[10] For the Watchman embolization rates were between 0.24%[11] and 1.3%.[12] In the Amulet IDE the device embolization was observed in 0.7% of the Amulet patients versus 0.2% of the Watchman 2.5 group.

The Watchman FLX was able to improve in terms of device embolization to between 0%[8,13,14] and 1.1%.[7] The improvement in terms of overall implantation success and device embolization rates for the Watchman FLX is likely attributable to the improved design particularly the two rows of J-anchors enabling full retrieval and repositioning of the device. The device is also more forgiving regarding sizing errors because the different device sizes have more of an overlap.

### Interference with Surrounding Structures

The LAA overlaps the pulmonary trunk anterosuperiorly, nearby a lateral ridge separating the ostium from the left upper pulmonary vein corresponding to the ligament of Marshall (posteriorly and superiorly), and the mitral valve, the left circumflex artery, and great cardiac vein (inferiorly). Given the lack of disk extending outside of the LAA orifice, endocardial single-lobe devices are theoretically less prone to jeopardize neighboring structures. In a preclinical model, Kar and colleagues[15] assessed the impact of LAAO on LAA adjacent structures using the Watchman and the Amplatzer Cardiac Plug (Abbott Vascular, Santa Clara, CA) devices. Watchman did not impinge the neighboring LAA structures, with tight apposition, sealing, and complete neoendothelialization at 28 days. Conversely, the disk of the Amplatzer Cardiac Plug could interfere with adjacent structures (extending beyond the pulmonary ridge or the posterior mitral valve annulus, leading to peridevice leak and left circumflex impingement in one case), resulting in delayed healing especially at the lower edge of the disk and end-screw hub regions, which could, in turn, potentially increase the risk of DRT formation. These findings highlight the importance of assessing pulmonary vein flow and mitral valve function during LAAO with lobe-and-disk devices. Also, although hypothesis-generating only, these data may be important to bear in mind when facing patients with large LAA (requiring the biggest devices) who have a short length between the left pulmonary superior vein and the mitral valve, which may particularly benefit

from single-lobe devices to avoid disk interference during the implantation (Fig. 2).

### Device-Related Thrombus

The reported rate of DRT following LAAO ranges between 0% and 17%, with a mean incidence of 3.8%, with wide variations depending on post-procedural antithrombotic regimen, device design, and surveillance imaging protocols.[16] Direct, randomized, head-to-head comparison between different devices is generally lacking, but data from large-scale meta-analysis has not shown any difference in DRT formation between single-lobe and disk-and-lobe devices. In a systematic review by Lempereur and colleagues,[17] DRT events were similar for the Watchman and Amplatzer devices (3.4% vs 4.6%, respectively), with large profile pin connectors or screws being associated with increased risk of thrombus. In a meta-analysis comparing the Watchman and Amplatzer devices (n = 614), DRT rates did not significantly differ between both devices.[18] Likewise, in a large meta-analysis including more than 12,000 patients from 66 studies, Alkhouli and colleagues[16] reported similar incidence of DRT between the ACP/Amulet and the Watchman device (3.6% vs 3.1%; $P = .24$). The AMULET-IDE (NCT02879448), has now reported similar DRT rates between Amulet and Watchman 2.5 (3.3% vs 4.5%).[9] The ongoing SWISS-APERO (NCT03399851) trial, directly comparing both devices in a randomized fashion, will also provide valuable information on this matter.

The Watchman device is the most widely used and studied single-lobe LAAO device so far. The incidence of DRT with Watchman has varied from 1.0% to 5.7%.[19] Rates of DRT with the earlier Watchman 2.5 version were slightly higher than those recently reported with the latest Watchman FLX device. In the PROTECT-AF trial, the observed rate of DRT was 5.7%, despite using an aggressive post-procedural antithrombotic regimen (6 weeks of aspirin plus warfarin followed by dual antiplatelet therapy until 6 months).[20] In the EWOLUTION registry, the mean DRT rate was 3.7%, with no association with the type of antithrombotic regimen.[21] In the Watchman FLX version, the delivery cable screw has been recessed with the aim to reduce the rate of DRT. Although the rate of DRT in the first multicenter experience with FLX was similar to the previous generation device (4.7%, very high-risk population, one-third discharged on single antiplatelet therapy),[8] the incidence of DRT in the PINNACLE FLX was markedly less (1.8% at 12 months).[13] Of note, all patients

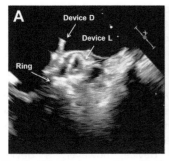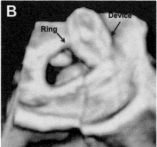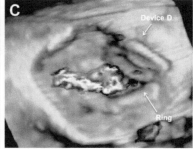

Fig. 2. Mitral valve erosion with the disk of an Amplatzer Amulet device. (A) Transesophageal echocardiogram showing device disk (D) protruding into the LAA and overriding the mitral valve ring. (B) Three-dimensional reconstruction with the disk protruding over the mitral ring. (C) Three-dimensional reconstruction with color reveals a severe mitral regurgitation.

were discharged on direct oral anticoagulant and aspirin (6 weeks), which may have influenced those findings. However, new flow assessment imaging techniques might be useful to identify those areas of the device with low-velocity flows that are more prone to developing DRT (Fig. 3–5).

Data regarding DRT formation with other single-lobe devices remain scarce. The reported rates of DRT with the Occlutech platform were approximately 6% in the first-in-man experience (2/30) and in the Occlutech LAA trial (4/66).[22] In a preclinical study with the latest generation Occlutech LAA Plus device, complete neoendothelium with no device thrombosis were observed at 3 months, despite no changes on the ball-shaped connection hub design.[23] The latter findings, and whether a more coaxial implantation with its steerable sheath will positively

impact on the risk of DRT are yet to be confirmed in clinical practice.

The rates of DRT following LAAO with Wavecrest have been low (<1%), with no DRT events observed in the WAVECREST I study.[24] The low thrombogenicity of the Wavecrest device has been attributed to the ePTFE properties, retraction of the center hub within the ePTFE fabric leaving no metal behind the left atrium, altogether resulting in a rapid surface endothelialization in preclinical models. The WACECREST 2 trial (NCT03302494), comparing the Wavecrest with the Watchman device, will provide further clinical information of the potential benefits of this single-lobe device.

## Residual Leaks

Peridevice leak is not uncommon after LAA closure. During the process of LAA closure there are three main causes of residual leak.

During the preimplantation phase, the LAA is sized using fluoroscopy and transesophageal echocardiogram to determine the device size and the LAA anatomy. The chosen device may not be adequate for the anatomy, oversized or undersized, and the final device choice may miss a lobe or offer incomplete coverage causing peridevice leak. During the implantation phase malapposition, deployment at the wrong depth, or not enough tissue capture with epicardial devices can cause peridevice leaks. Postprocedurally migration of device or suture or incomplete endothelialization can cause peridevice leak.

The incidence of peridevice leak varies depending on the definition and the imaging modalities used. Further complicating a comparison are varying definitions of leaks depending on which device type was used for closure.[25] When defining peridevice leak, both randomized trials using the Watchman device[26] have

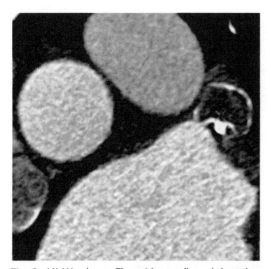

Fig. 3. (A) Watchman Flex with an adhered thrombus in the left atrial side. (B) Thrombus resolution after 3 months of therapy with low-molecular heparin.

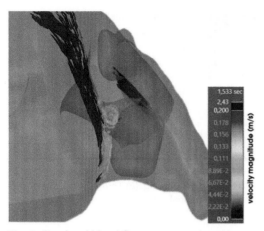

Fig. 4. Simulated blood flow patterns colored by velocity magnitude (*blue* is low velocity <0.10 m/second and *red* is high velocity >0.20 m/second). A slow flow pattern is observed on the device close to the pulmonary ridge.

The incidence of peridevice leak varies a lot depending on the study ranging from 7% at 7 months of which 2% were relevant[28] to a study with 32% at 12 months of which 12% were relevant leaks.[29] A postinterventional nonrandomized computed tomography study, however, showed peridevice leaks in 68.5% of patients with a reduction to 56.7% at the 1-year follow-up. This was a small study where no relevant difference could be found between the Amulet and the Watchman device; however, a device compression of less than 10% was associated with the occurrence of leaks.[30] In the Amulet IDE study the Amulet device showed to be superior in the reduction of residual leaks, with 98.9% of Amulet patients without significant residual jet (≤5 mm) versus 96.8% in the Watchman group.[9] These differences might be related to the edge effect described with the Watchman 2.5 device. Even if the device is perfectly upsized to get a good contact on all sides, with atrial remodeling a small leak can develop later in the clinical course on the edges, creating the edge effect. This variation in tissue remodeling around the edge of the device probably explains the shift in the size and location of the leak in percutaneous LAAO devices.[11]

Overall, the clinical relevance of peridevice leaks still is not well understood. There are indications that peridevice leak may be related to an increased incidence of stroke; however, patients who are found to have a relevant leak are usually kept on oral anticoagulation or receive leak closure. The Munich

defined a relevant (severe) leak to be more than 5 mm in transesophageal echocardiogram (moderate, 1–3 mm; minor, <1 mm). In contrast, a peridevice leak for the ACP or Amulet is defined as flow around the device lobe with greater than 5 mm being severe, 3 to 5 mm moderate, and 1 to 3 mm mild.[27] In both devices a leak is defined as flow behind the device. However, the Amulet has room in between the lobe and the disk and residual blood flow in this area may also contribute as a possible source for embolization of thrombus.

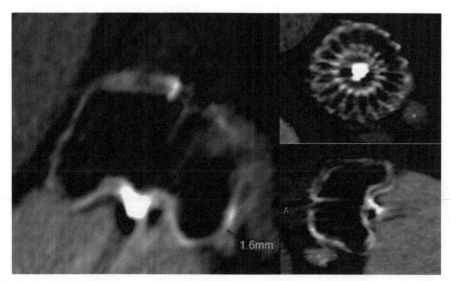

Fig. 5. Watchman FLX device with a small peridevice leak (1.6 mm) diagnosed by cardiac computed tomography angiogram.

consensus paper recognizes that current definitions for peridevice leak are not adequate and aims to create a pathway of how to assess leaks.[31] Until there are comparative data between the two different types of devices no clear conclusion can be reached as to which approach may be superior or which patients may profit more from one than the other.

The development of the Watchman FLX aims to reduce the incidence of peridevice leak through the addition of more struts with the aim of creating more contact points between the occluder and the LAA ostium. The increased covering of now two-thirds of the Watchman FLX occluder aims to allow for a more off axis implantation while still sealing of the LAA. In the PINNACLE FLX study the new generation Watchman Flex device showed the lowest safety event rate was of 0.5% (combination of death, ischemic stroke, systemic embolism, or device- or procedure-related events requiring open cardiac surgery or major endovascular intervention, such as pseudoaneurysm repair, arteriovenous fistula repair, or another major endovascular repair), the lowest observed in any prior Watchman study. Moreover, in this series the incidence of any peridevice flow with jet size greater than 5 mm was of 0% at 12 months, revealing a real impact in the design change of the device.[13]

## SUMMARY

Two main philosophies have predominated in the design of LAAO devices: the lobe-disk (pacifier) and the single-lobe (plug). The main advantage of the pacifier is related to a wider possibility of covering all sorts of appendage anatomies, using the lobe as an anchoring system while the disk serves to seal the appendage. However, the disk might be unnecessary in standard anatomies, and might interfere with surrounding structures instead. Moreover, when the disk protrudes into the LAA, this might favor device thrombosis. In this regard, single-lobe devices have the main advantage that none of the device protrudes into the LAA, and therefore there is no risk of interference. The Watchman FLX device has improved the capacity of the device to cover all sorts of appendage anatomies with a really forgiving and stable device. The initial experience has revealed a high implantation success and low embolization rates, good sealing, and has not increased DRT.

The aim of LAAO devices is to be able to cover a wide range of appendage anatomies, to get perfect sealing (no leak) with stability (no embolization), without getting thrombus on the device itself (DRT). In this regard, no significant differences have been observed between the two main representatives of the pacifier (Amulet) and plug philosophy (Watchman FLX).

Results from head-to-head comparisons will be published soon, which will allow more knowledge about outcomes and a better understanding of each device.

## CLINICS CARE POINTS

- An adequate imaging study to assess left atrial appendage anatomy is recommended to select the proper device for occlusion.
- The aim of the procedure is to have a perfect seal of the appendage to avoid future complications that might have a clinical impact.
- After occlusion adequate follow-up with imaging should be mandatory, to discard DRT, peridevice leak, and other potential complications.
- Cardiac computed tomography should be favored as an imaging technique, because it is more sensible to assess peridevice leak and gives more information about the disposition of the device in the appendage.

## DISCLOSURE

DA is a proctor for Boston Scientific and Abbott.

## REFERENCES

1. García-Fernández MA, Pérez-David E, Quiles J, et al. Role of left atrial appendage obliteration in stroke reduction in patients with mitral valve prosthesis: a transesophageal echocardiographic study. J Am Coll Cardiol 2003;42(7):1253–8.
2. Haïssaguerre M, Jaïs P, Shah DC, et al. Spontaneous initiation of atrial fibrillation by ectopic beats originating in the pulmonary veins. N Engl J Med 1998;339(10):659–66.
3. Sievert H, Lesh MD, Trepels T, et al. Percutaneous left atrial appendage transcatheter occlusion to prevent stroke in high-risk patients with atrial fibrillation: early clinical experience. Circulation 2002; 105(16):1887–9.
4. Freixa X, Cepas-Guillen P, Flores-Umanzor E, et al. Pulmonary ridge coverage and device-related

thrombosis after left atrial appendage occlusion. Eurointervention 2021;16(15):e1288–94.

5. Berti S, Santoro G, Brscic E, et al. Left atrial appendage closure using AMPLATZER™ devices: a large, multicenter, Italian registry. Int J Cardiol 2017;248:103–7.

6. Landmesser U, Tondo C, Camm J, et al. Left atrial appendage occlusion with the AMPLATZER Amulet device: one-year follow-up from the prospective global Amulet observational registry. Eurointervention J Eur Collab Work Gr Interv Cardiol Eur Soc Cardiol 2018;14(5):e590–7.

7. Ledwoch J, Franke J, Akin I, et al. WATCHMAN versus ACP or Amulet devices for left atrial appendage occlusion: a sub-analysis of the multicentre LAARGE registry. Eurointervention J Eur Collab Work Gr Interv Cardiol Eur Soc Cardiol 2020;16(11):e942–9.

8. Cruz-González I, Korsholm K, Trejo-Velasco B, et al. Procedural and short-term results with the new Watchman FLX left atrial appendage occlusion device. JACC Cardiovasc Interv 2020;13(23):2732–41.

9. Lakkireddy D, Thaler D, Ellis CR, et al. Amplatzer™ Amulet™ left atrial appendage occluder versus Watchman™ device for stroke prophylaxis (amulet ide): a randomized controlled trial. Circulation 2021;144(19):1543–52. https://doi.org/10.1161/CIRCULATIONAHA.121.057063.

10. Nietlispach F, Gloekler S, Krause R, et al. Amplatzer left atrial appendage occlusion: single center 10-year experience. Catheter Cardiovasc Interv 2013; 82(2):283–9.

11. Pillarisetti J, Reddy YM, Gunda S, et al. Endocardial (Watchman) vs epicardial (Lariat) left atrial appendage exclusion devices: understanding the differences in the location and type of leaks and their clinical implications. Hear Rhythm 2015;12(7): 1501–7.

12. Reddy VY, Gibson DN, Kar S, et al. Post-approval U.S. experience with left atrial appendage closure for stroke prevention in atrial fibrillation. J Am Coll Cardiol 2017;69(3):253–61.

13. Kar S, Doshi SK, Sadhu A, et al. Primary outcome evaluation of a next-generation left atrial appendage closure device: results from the PINNACLE FLX Trial. Circulation 2021;143(18): 1754–62.

14. Korsholm K, Samaras A, Andersen A, et al. The Watchman FLX device: first European experience and feasibility of intracardiac echocardiography to guide implantation. JACC Clin Electrophysiol 2020;6(13):1633–42.

15. Kar S, Hou D, Jones R, et al. Impact of Watchman and Amplatzer devices on left atrial appendage adjacent structures and healing response in a canine model. JACC Cardiovasc Interv 2014;7(7):801–9.

16. Alkhouli M, Busu T, Shah K, et al. Incidence and clinical impact of device-related thrombus following percutaneous left atrial appendage occlusion: a meta-analysis. JACC Clin Electrophysiol 2018;4(12):1629–37.

17. Lempereur M, Aminian A, Freixa X, et al. Device-associated thrombus formation after left atrial appendage occlusion: a systematic review of events reported with the Watchman, the Amplatzer Cardiac Plug and the Amulet. Catheter Cardiovasc Interv 2017;90(5):E111–21.

18. Basu Ray I, Khanra D, Shah S, et al. Meta-analysis comparing Watchman(TM) and Amplatzer devices for stroke prevention in atrial fibrillation. Frontiers in cardiovascular medicine 2020;7:89.

19. Asmarats L, Rodés-Cabau J. Percutaneous left atrial appendage closure: current devices and clinical outcomes. Circ Cardiovasc Interv 2017;10(11).

20. Main ML, Fan D, Reddy VY, et al. Assessment of device-related thrombus and associated clinical outcomes with the WATCHMAN left atrial appendage closure device for embolic protection in patients with atrial fibrillation (from the PROTECT-AF Trial). Am J Cardiol 2016;117(7):1127–34.

21. Boersma LV, Ince H, Kische S, et al. Efficacy and safety of left atrial appendage closure with WATCHMAN in patients with or without contraindication to oral anticoagulation: 1-year follow-up outcome data of the EWOLUTION trial. Hear Rhythm 2017;14(9):1302–8.

22. Bellmann B, Schnupp S, Kühnlein P, et al. Left atrial appendage closure with the new Occlutech® device: first in man experience and neurological outcome. J Cardiovasc Electrophysiol 2017;28(3): 315–20.

23. Reinthaler M, Grosshauser J, Schmidt T, et al. Preclinical assessment of a modified Occlutech left atrial appendage closure device in a porcine model. Sci Rep 2021;11(1):2988.

24. Gianni C, Anannab A, Sahore Salwan A, et al. Closure of the left atrial appendage using percutaneous transcatheter occlusion devices. J Cardiovasc Electrophysiol 2020;31(8):2179–86.

25. Sahore A, Della Rocca DG, Anannab A, et al. Clinical implications and management strategies for left atrial appendage leaks. Card Electrophysiol Clin 2020;12(1):89–96.

26. Reddy VY, Doshi SK, Kar S, et al. 5-year outcomes after left atrial appendage closure: from the PREVAIL and PROTECT AF Trials. J Am Coll Cardiol 2017;70(24):2964–75.

27. Saw J, Tzikas A, Shakir S, et al. Incidence and clinical impact of device-associated thrombus and peri-device leak following left atrial appendage closure with the Amplatzer cardiac plug. JACC Cardiovasc Interv 2017;10(4):391–9.

28. Viles-Gonzalez JF, Kar S, Douglas P, et al. The clinical impact of incomplete left atrial appendage closure with the Watchman Device in patients with atrial fibrillation: a PROTECT AF (Percutaneous Closure of the Left Atrial Appendage Versus Warfarin Therapy for Prevention of Stroke in Patients Wi. J Am Coll Cardiol 2012;59(10):923–9.

29. Raphael CE, Friedman PA, Saw J, et al. Residual leaks following percutaneous left atrial appendage occlusion: assessment and management implications. Eurointervention 2017;13(10):1218–25.

30. Nguyen A, Gallet R, Riant E, et al. Peridevice leak after left atrial appendage closure: incidence, risk factors, and clinical impact. Can J Cardiol 2019;35(4):405–12.

31. Tzikas A, Holmes DRJ, Gafoor S, et al. Percutaneous left atrial appendage occlusion: the Munich consensus document on definitions, endpoints, and data collection requirements for clinical studies. Europace 2017;19(1):4–15.

# The Strengths and Weaknesses of Left Atrial Appendage Ligation or Exclusion (LARIAT, AtriaClip, Surgical Suture)

Randall J. Lee, MD, PhD[a],*, Thorsten Hanke, MD[b]

---

**KEYWORDS**

- Epicardial LAA exclusion • Surgical LAA closure • Suture • AtriClip • LARIAT

---

**KEY POINTS**

- Surgical LAA exclusion has been performed for more than 60 years either during mitral valve surgery and coronary artery bypass grafting, or as an integral part of the Cox maze procedure for atrial fibrillation (AF).
- AHA/ACC/ESC guidelines for treatment of valvular heart disease recommend exclusion of the LAA during concomitant procedures as a prophylactic measure to eliminate a primary source of thrombus (Class I indication).
- The LAAOS III prospective randomized trial demonstrates that surgical epicardial exclusion of the LAA reduces ischemic stroke or systemic embolism.
- Initial observational studies and registries suggest that percutaneous LAA ligation with the LARIAT device is safe and effectively eliminates the LAA. Results of the prospective randomized aMAZE trial will validate the safety and effectiveness of LAA closure.

---

## BACKGROUND

Atrial fibrillation (AF) is the most common arrhythmia observed in clinical practice. The number of patients with AF is likely to increase 2.5-fold in the next 50 years, reflecting a growing and aging population at risk.[1] The AF population has a higher risk of morbidity and mortality associated with an increased incidence of other heart disease (eg, heart failure, stroke).[2] Hospitalizations are more common in patients with AF than patients without AF and add an estimated $26 billion to the US health care bill annually.[2] Ectopic foci within the pulmonary veins (PVs) are the most active drivers of AF; however, other non-PV drivers may contribute to the initiation and maintenance of advanced forms of AF. These ectopic non-PV foci contribute more to nonparoxysmal AF and can be located in the superior vena cava, ligament of Marshall, coronary sinus, crista terminalis, left atrial (LA) posterior wall, or the left atrial appendage (LAA).[3,4] The LAA specifically has been implicated in both the persistence of AF and the source of thrombus formation, attributed to stasis of blood flow in the appendage itself.[5]

AF increases a patient's risk of ischemic (or embolic) stroke 5-fold.[6,7] In fact, AF is responsible for up to 20% of all strokes with a mean annualized stroke rate of 4.0% per year.[8–10] At least two-thirds of the ischemic cerebrovascular events and half of all vascular events in patients

---

[a] Cardiac Electrophysiology, University of California, San Francisco, 500 Parnassus Avenue, Box 1354, San Francisco, CA 94143, USA; [b] Department of Cardiovascular Surgery, ASKLEPIOS Klinikum Harburg, Abteilung Herzchirurgie, Eißendorfer Pferdeweg 52, 21075 Hamburg, Germany
* Corresponding author.
*E-mail address:* Randall.Lee@ucsf.edu

Intervent Cardiol Clin 11 (2022) 205–217
https://doi.org/10.1016/j.iccl.2022.01.001
2211-7458/22/© 2022 Elsevier Inc. All rights reserved.

with nonvalvular AF are related to the left atrial (LA) thrombi.[8,11,12] Ninety percent of the LA thrombi found in patients with nonvalvular AF occurred in the LAA, whereas only 57% of valvular AF were located in the LAA.[13] Embolic stroke secondary to AF is associated with a mortality of greater than 30% at 1 year.[14,15]

The LAA is a trabecular pouch extending from the LA. This structure has been associated with various pathologic conditions.[3,16–18] Surgical LAA exclusion has been performed for more than 60 years either during mitral valve surgery and coronary artery bypass grafting or as an integral part of the Cox-Maze procedure for AF.[19–23] The 2006 American Heart Association/American College of Cardiology/European Society of Cardiology (AHA/ACC/ESC) guidelines for treatment of AF, 2014 AHA/ACC/ESC guidelines for management of patients with AF, and the AHA/ACC/ESC guidelines for treatment of valvular heart disease recommend exclusion of the LAA during concomitant procedures as a prophylactic measure to eliminate a primary source of thrombus.[2,24–26] The 2012 ESC Guidelines for AF management also notes that LAA occlusion should be considered in patients with thromboembolic risk and cannot be managed with long-term oral anticoagulant (OAC).[27] These are class IIB recommendations with level B and C evidence. The 2014 NICE Guidelines recommend that LAA closure be considered for contraindicated or intolerant patients.[28]

With more than 60 years of history, the clinical basis for ligation and exclusion of the LAA has been firmly established. Numerous approaches have been used for surgical LAA exclusion, including surgical resections, suture ligation, cutting and noncutting staples, percutaneous implants, and surgical clips. The surgical techniques, both epicardial and endocardial approaches, for LAA exclusion include simple neck ligation, purse-string techniques, vascular stapling methods or endocardial suture ligation, and sometimes LAA excision. There is no consensus of the best method, and most of the published literature consists of retrospective analyses. The surgical goal in LAA is obliteration of "our most lethal human attachment," and its potential for future thrombus formation.[29] Although recommended by guidelines, LAA exclusion does not always occur because of incomplete closure and adverse event concerns. Complete LAA ligation has been shown to be more effective, during mitral valve replacement, in the reduction of late embolism than incomplete ligation.[30] The LAA tissue is frail and easily damaged. As a result, along with its anatomic

position next to coronary vessels, tissue tears and bleeding are crucial surgical risks.[31] In addition, residual leaks may occur from either suture or staplers and is dependent on the operator's technique and experience.

Endocardial suture ligation of the LAA is an extremely invasive procedure requiring the use of cardiopulmonary bypass and invasion of the atrial dome with associated risk of bleeding and injury to the circumflex coronary artery owing to its proximity to the LAA. In addition, endocardial suture ligation has been shown to be incomplete in 10% to 30% of patients.[32–34] This high rate of incomplete closure is attributed to several factors: the procedure is performed when the heart is in a flaccid state, the access is generally awkward for traditional suturing, and there is no ready method to confirm completeness of closure intraoperatively. The closure result can be adequately assessed only after the heart is reperfused, after the opportunity to rectify incomplete closure has passed.

Epicardial suture ligation of the LAA can also be performed without opening the LA and without cardiopulmonary bypass.[35] Epicardial suture closure of the LAA is conventionally performed by either directly sewing the appendage closed or tightening pretied suture loops around the base of the LAA. The success of complete epicardial suture closure ranges from 23% to 100% and is both technique and operator dependent.[36–38] Incomplete suture ligation of the LAA does not appear to be a degenerative process (such as owing to suture dehiscence), but rather is present immediately after the procedure. Complications rarely arise because of suture closure of the LAA and are generally limited to LAA tearing that occurs either during the suture needle placement or while grasping the LAA as is required in conventional open surgical approaches, and has been reported between 7% and 25%.[29,35,37]

Kanderian and colleagues[36] described a retrospective study observing various LAA closure techniques. From 2546 patients with surgical LAA closure, they reviewed 137 patients with a postoperative transesophageal echocardiogram (TEE; mean time, 8.1 ± 12 months). Among the patients were those who underwent excision (52 patients), suture exclusion (73 patients), or stapler without excision (12 patients). The investigators defined successful closure as no persistent color Doppler flow jet by TEE and a remnant LAA stump less than 1 cm. There was a complete closure rate of 40% (55/137 overall; excision: 38/52, suture: 17/73, stapler: 0/12). At the time of their follow-up, patients with TEE were asked if they experienced a stroke or transient ischemic attack (TIA) since the time of the procedure. There was an 11% (6/55) rate in those with complete LAA closure as compared with the 15% (12/82) rate in those with unsuccessful LAA closure; however, the investigators caution whether residual flow or remnant stump is truly associated with an increased risk of emboli.

## EPICARDIAL EXCLUSION OF THE LEFT ATRIAL APPENDAGE

The original surgical approaches to "curative" procedures for AF included LAA exclusion.[22,39] A study of 178 patients with AF that had OAC discontinued after a Cox-Maze III procedure found no strokes over 10 years.[39] The 2006 AHA/ACC/ESC guidelines for treatment of AF, 2014 AHA/ACC/ESC guidelines for management of patients with AF, and the AHA/ACC/ESC guidelines for treatment of valvular heart disease recommend exclusion of the LAA during concomitant procedures as a prophylactic measure to eliminate a primary source of thrombus.[2,24–26] Exclusion of the LAA in conjunction with pulmonary vein isolation (PVI) catheter ablation would best emulate the gold-standard Cox-Maze AF treatment and potentially provide similar prevention of embolic events and remove a contributor to AF. Two epicardial LAA exclusion devices are currently being used. The AtriClip is performed either concomitantly with open-heart surgery or thoracoscopically, whereas the LARIAT procedure is a percutaneous approach for epicardial LAA exclusion.

## THE AtriClip LEFT ATRIAL APPENDAGE EXCLUSION DEVICE

The AtriClip device (AtriCure, Inc, Mason, OH, USA) is the first approved device for surgical LAA exclusion. The AtriClip device has 510(k) Food and Drug Administration clearance for LAA closure in patients undergoing cardiac surgery and has been deployed in more than 300,000 patients worldwide. The AtriClip device is a self-closing, implantable clip made of 2 parallel titanium bars connected with nitinol hinges covered in a braided polyester lining. The clip is attached to a disposable applicator. The clip may be repositioned if initial placement is inadequate. Once closed, the AtriClip device produces a constant compression pressure, assuring complete exclusion of the LAA. Early animal studies demonstrated that the clip left a smooth, linear occlusion line without laceration

and did not migrate or damage adjacent structures.[40–42] The animal studies also supported that the LAA tissue, distal to the clip, atrophied (after 30-day follow-up) and was replaced with fibrous tissues.

The first human trial treated 34 patients, median age 71 ± 10 years, with the AtriClip device placed during concomitant AF ablation and open-heart cardiac surgery.[43] The clip was maneuvered to the base of the LAA while the surgeon immobilized the heart and applied it successfully in a single attempt. Patients on cardiopulmonary bypass had the clip applied before opening the aortic cross-clamp. Those patients off-pump had their clip applied after revascularization with sufficient coronary perfusion. There were no device-related complications, but there was an operative mortality of 8.8% (n = 3; iatrogenic lung bleed, hepatic failure, and aortic tear). Those that completed computed tomography (CT) at 3-month follow-up demonstrated LAA exclusion. The exclusions did not affect LA diameter or left ventricular function.

The feasibility and efficacy prospective, multicenter closure study, the Exclusion of Left Atrial Appendage with AtriClip Exclusion Device in Patients Undergoing Concomitant Cardiac Surgery (EXCLUDE), enrolled 71 patients undergoing concomitant open cardiac surgery.[44] The mean age was 73.3 years, and 38.0% (n = 27) had a CHADS$_2$ score greater than 2. The clip was successfully deployed in 95.7% (67/70) of patients with a residual appendage stump left in 3 subjects. The LAA, pulmonary artery, and circumflex artery were not damaged in any patients during the procedure. There was 98.2% successful LAA closure verified as verified by CT (55/56) or TEE (5/5) at the 3-month follow-up. There were no serious adverse events related to the device or clip placement procedure that occurred within 30 days of the procedure. Two (3.1%, 2/64) late neurologic events, 1 TIA and 1 stroke, occurred during the 12-month follow-up. This initial study has been corroborated by other single-center observational studies.[45–50]

A 65-patient retrospective analysis assessed the long-term LAA efficacy of the AtriClip device applied via a totally thorascopic approach with CT scanning.[51] In this retrospective analysis, subjects underwent CT angiography ≥90 days after implantation that was independently assessed by a radiologist. Complete LAA closure (defined by complete exclusion of the LAA with no exposed trabeculations, and clip within 1 cm from the left circumflex artery) was found in 61/65 subjects (93.9%). Two clips were placed too distally, leaving a large stump with exposed trabeculae. Two clips failed to address a secondary lobe. No major complications were associated with thoracoscopic placement of the AtriClip device. Follow-up over 183 patient-years revealed 1 stroke in a patient with complete closure and no thrombus.

A recent meta-analysis of the safety and efficacy of the AtriClip device (placed thoracoscopically or during open concomitant surgery) found that in 922 patients acute closure was 97.8%, and there were no periprocedural device-related adverse events.[52] Stroke rates ranged from 0.2 to 1.5 per 100 patient-years in follow-up, with 59% of patients able to discontinue anticoagulation.

The AtriClip device portfolio has evolved from the original closed-ended clip to include an open-ended V-clip. The AtriClip devices perform identically, and device selection is solely based on surgeon preference. The V-Clip can be applied directly to the base of the LAA, has a smaller profile than the original AtriClip device, and has an applier that facilitates one-hand device placement. The first-generation closed-ended AtriClip device is favored by surgeons who prefer to pass the clip over the LAA to capture its entirety, then move the device to the base. Both generations of AtriClip devices have appliers to facilitate use in sternotomy and minimally invasive surgical approaches.

## LARIAT LEFT ATRIAL APPENDAGE EXCLUSION SYSTEM

The concept for the LARIAT LAA Exclusion System was originally developed to provide a percutaneous, minimally invasive epicardial approach to LAA closure with the advantage of eliminating the need for a permanent implant inside the LAA. The LARIAT LAA exclusion system allows for positioning and deployment of an epicardial ligature on the base of the LAA. The LARIAT LAA exclusion system consists of the LARIAT suture delivery device, endocardial and epicardial magnet wires, an endocardial balloon catheter, a tension device, and a suture cutter.[53,54] The first LARIAT device was CE-marked in 2009. Since then, several variants of the LARIAT LAA exclusion system have received CE-marking for LAA closure and 510(k) clearance in the United States for soft tissue approximation and closure.

Ligation of the LAA base results in discontinuation of blood perfusion of the distal LAA tissue and initiates ischemic necrosis of the appendage.[55–57] Within a 90-day period, the tissue compression of the ligation results in complete exclusion of the LAA as it atrophies and resorbs.[55] Initially, the ligature mechanically excludes the LAA by approximating the walls of the ostium of the LAA, which leads to ischemic necrosis of the LAA myocardial tissue. The ischemic tissue distal to the ligature becomes nonviable and inexcitable (ie, cannot electrically create or conduct action potentials). The LAA ostium becomes occluded and over time is sealed with smooth fibrous tissue, which subsequently endothelializes. This results in complete and permanent mechanical exclusion and electrical isolation because the distal LAA after ligation is devoid of electrically excitable myocardial cells and eventually resorbs and disappears. The tightened ligature causes the LAA to atrophy and resorb over time.[54,55] The epicardial LAA exclusion leads to mechanical closure of the LAA, thus preventing thrombus formation,[58] as well electrical isolation of the LAA, debulking of the LA, and favorable electrical remodeling of the LA.[59–62]

The LARIAT LAA Exclusion System was initially designed and first used in humans in 2009.[63] This was followed by a clinical trial to assess efficacy and safety of the LARIAT system for LAA ligation.[53] The suture implant and suture knot that excludes the LAA have not changed since 2009. More than 8000 LARIAT devices (AtriCure, Inc, Mason, OH, USA) have been used worldwide over the past 12 years. There have been changes in the LARIAT suture delivery device since its inception in 2009. The LARIAT+ has improved features consisting of the following: (1) expansion of the snare from 40 mm to 45 mm, (2) addition of a platinum-iridium "L" marker that allows for easier identification of the correct orientation of the LARIAT+ snare loop under fluoroscopy, (3) a stainless steel wire braid on catheter shaft that provides improved "torque-ability" of the catheter with 1:1 torque control for ease of positioning during LAA capture.[64] More recently, the LARIAT RS has a releasable and fully retractable snare feature added to the LARIAT+ device to increase the ease of removal from the tissue after suture deployment. Further development is in progress for an epicardial only LAA ligation LARIAT system.[65]

The LARIAT LAA Exclusion System was used in a single-center observational trial that demonstrated the safe delivery of the suture to close the LAA in 85 of 89 (96%) treated patients.[53] Ninety-six percent (85/89) had successful LAA ligation, with complete acute closure (defined as <1-mm jet) in 82 patients and ≤3-mm jet in

3 patients. At 90 days, 95% (77/81) of patients had complete closure, with 4 patients having jets ≤3 mm. At 1 year, complete closure was 98% (64/65), with 1 patient having a jet ≤2 mm. There were no device-related complications. Three pericardial- or transseptal access-related complications occurred (2 cardiac perforations and 1 arterial vessel perforation). One patient had a late pericardial effusion at 2 weeks requiring pericardiocentesis, and 1 patient developed a thrombus lateral to the ligation site that resolved with oral anticoagulation therapy.

Several subsequent small observational studies corroborated the feasibility and safety of the LARIAT to effective and safely exclude the LAA.[66,67] However, the initial expanded use of the LARIAT device demonstrated continued acceptable LAA closure results, but with higher bleeding and adverse rates.[68,69] Subsequently, experience, training, and the adoption of a micropuncture needle to reduce right ventricular (RV) perforations and colchicine treatment to mitigate postligation pericardial effusions were incorporated in the LARIAT procedure. The use of the micropuncture needle and colchicine has helped to mitigate complications and major bleeding episodes.[54,70] A large, multicenter, observational study of 712 patients treated at 18 US centers with the LAA Exclusion System further demonstrated the safety and performance of the LARIAT System.[71] Successful ligation was achieved in 96% (682/712) of patients attempted. Acute closure rate was 98.1% (669/682) with 13 patients having less than 2-mm leak. At 1 to 3 months, 1 out of 480 patients had a leak greater than 5 mm (0.2%), 31 (6.5%) had leaks 2 to 5 mm, and 448 (93%) had complete closure. The acute complication rate was 5.3%, with 1 (0.14%) mortality. Further verification of the effectiveness and safety of the LARIAT procedure was demonstrated in an independent multicenter European registry of 141 patients with nonvalvular AF and contraindication to oral anticoagulation.[72] Acute LAA exclusion was achieved in 138/141 patients (97.9%). Complete LAA closure or leaks less than 2 mm were seen in 78.6% of patients. LAA leaks of between 2 and 5 mm were seen in 18.4% of patients. Only 3 patients (2.9%) had leaks greater than 5 mm. However, follow-up TEE did not reveal any leaks greater than 5 mm. Three patients (2.1%) did not undergo attempted deployment of the LARIAT device because of pericardial adhesion. Serious periprocedural adverse events occurred in 2.8% (4/141)

patients. There were no deaths attributed to the procedure or LARIAT device.

## SALIENT EFFECTS OF EPICARDIAL LEFT ATRIAL APPENDAGE EXCLUSION

### Epicardial Left Atrial Appendage Exclusion for Prevention of Thrombus Formation

The LAA is a complex structure of variable morphology derived from the embryonic LA. The endocardium of the LAA adds to the anatomic complexity with the heterogeneous network of pectinate muscle. The extensive arborized structure is thought to encourage thrombus formation and increased risk of stroke independent of blood stasis.[73] A significantly higher prothrombotic state as reflected by elevated thrombin generation markers (F1 + 2 prothrombin fragments) and D-dimer[74–76] and a prolonged clot lysis time[74] have been observed in patients with AF. An initial study has demonstrated that there is a significant prolongation of clot lysis time from LAA blood samples and a significant reduction of LAA clot porosity compared with peripheral blood,[77] suggesting that the LAA is a prothrombotic structure. The local prothrombotic state may contribute to LAA thrombus formation and device-related thrombi. It has been widely debated if LAA closure could be an alternative to pharmacologic treatment for stroke prevention.[11] As early as the 1940s, the LAA was excluded during mitral valve surgeries to prevent thromboembolic events.[22,78,79]

Observational studies have suggested a stroke prevention benefit with epicardial exclusion of the LAA. In a multicenter registry, 291 AtriClip devices were deployed epicardially in patients undergoing open-heart surgery.[80] The mean CHA2DS2-VASc score was 3.1 ± 1.5. Patients were followed for a mean of 36 ± 23 months (range, 1–97 months). OAC were discontinued in 57% of patients (166 of 291 patients). There was an 87.5% relative risk reduction of embolic events with an ischemic stroke rate of 0.5 per 100 patient-years compared with a similar CHADS-VASc score cohort that has an expected stroke rate of 4/0 per 100 patient-years. In the subgroup treated with OAC therapy, there were no strokes. The excellent LAA closure rate of the of the AtriClip devices enhances its ability for preventing LAA thrombus formation.

A prospective multicenter observational study in 139 patients with a contraindication to OAC therapy and undergoing LAA ligation with the LARIAT suture delivery device had a composite event rate of stroke and systemic embolism of

1.0% per year at a mean follow-up of 2.9 years.[58] The stroke and systemic embolism rate of 1.0% per year in this LARIAT population represented an 84% reduction in risk compared with a cohort with a similar CHADs-VASc score. Postprocedure LAA ligation antithrombotic regimen included no therapy (n = 44, 32%), aspirin (ASA; n = 83, 60%), clopidogrel (n = 3, 2%), ASA plus clopidogrel (n = 9, 6%). No patients received transition OAC therapy. Similar embolic event rates have been reported in subsequent registries with a post-LAA ligation thrombus formation of less than 2%.[68,71,72]

Recently, 2 prospective, multicenter randomized studies have evaluated LAA exclusion in the prevention of thromboembolic events during cardiac surgery (LAAOS III and ATLAS). The ATLAS trial was a prospective, randomized, multicenter feasibility trial that evaluated thromboembolic events and major bleeding rates with and without LAA exclusion in cardiac surgery patients who developed postoperative AF (POAF).[81] The cardiac surgery patients had a CHADS2-VASc score ≥2, an HAS-BLED score ≥2, and did not have preexisting AF. Patients were randomized in 2:1 AtriClip device to no AtriClip device and then followed for at least 1 year. Most of the patients were not on OAC therapy (24% for left atrial appendage exclusion group and 16% in no LAAE group; P = .33). There was a significant increase (P = .05%) in POAF in the LAAE group (47%) compared with the no LAAE group (38%). Successful LAAE was observed in 99.2% of the patients with 1 of 376 (0.03%) patients having a procedural serious adverse event. There was no significant difference in mortality between LAAE and no LAAE at 30 days and 1 year. In patients who developed POAF, there was an observed 51% reduction of thromboembolic events in the LAAE group (3.4%) compared with the no LAAE group (7.0%).

The LAAOS III trial tested the hypothesis that LAAE at the time of other cardiac surgery in patients with AF reduces ischemic stroke or systemic thromboembolic events.[82] The trial was a multicenter, randomized trial involving patients with AF and a CHA2DS2-VASc score ≥2 who were scheduled to undergo cardiac surgery for another indication.[82] The participants (N = 4811 patients) were assigned in a 1:1 randomization to undergo or not undergo exclusion of the LAA during surgery. The LAA exclusion techniques included stapler occlusion, amputation of the LAA with suture closure (preferred method), exclusion devices, endovascular suture closure, and other approved techniques. The participants received usual care, including oral anticoagulation, during follow-up (80%, 77%, and 75% OAC use in the LAAE group at 1- to 3-year follow-up and 79%, 78%, and 78% OAC use in the no LAAE group, respectively). The primary outcome at 3.8 years demonstrated that surgical LAAE reduces ischemic stroke or systemic embolism by 33% compared with no LAAE, and by 42% after the 30-day postoperative period. The benefit of LAAE was additive to OAC therapy. The incidence of perioperative bleeding, heart failure, or death did not differ significantly between the trial groups, indicating that there was not a significant tradeoff in safety with the added LAAE procedure.

## Left Atrial Remodeling

LAA epicardial exclusion results in debulking of the LA with a lasting reduction in LA volume,[62] which is an independent risk factor for AF or recurrence of AF after catheter ablation.[83,84] Favorable reverse electrical atrial remodeling as evidenced by changes in P-wave amplitude, P-wave duration, and P-wave dispersion is consistent with decreases in atrial mass, intraatrial conduction, and atrial dispersion that also favors maintenance of sinus rhythm.[60,61,85,86] Although PVI has been shown to favorably reverse remodel the LA,[85,86] the addition of LAA epicardial exclusion to PVI significantly adds further beneficial LA electrical remodeling.[87]

## Left Atrial Appendage Electrical Isolation

Epicardial exclusion of the LAA has been associated with electrical isolation.[59,88] Both the AtriClip device and the LARIAT have demonstrated LAA electrical isolation. LA, LAA, and RV pacing and sensing were performed in 10 patients undergoing open-heart surgery before and after epicardial clip exclusion of the LAA.[88] In all 10 patients, there was demonstration of inability to excite the LAA when pacing the LA after clip placement (entrance block) and block to the LA and the lack of acceleration to the RV ("exit block") when pacing the LAA. Electrical isolation of the LAA was investigated with the LARIAT device in 68 patients with contraindication or intolerance to oral anticoagulation therapy.[59] During a LARIAT procedure, patients had unipolar (n = 30) or bipolar (n = 38) LAA voltage measurements pre-LAA ligation and post-LAA ligation. A significant reduction of LAA voltage was observed with closure of the snare, and complete elimination of electrical activity with tightening of the suture in a third of the patients. After closure of the snare, pacing from the LAA did not capture the LA, demonstrating that electrical propagation from the LAA to the LA was eliminated. Because the LAA undergoes necrosis and atrophy after LAA ligation,[56,57] the electrical isolation of the LAA is permanent.

Direct effects of electrical isolation of the LAA arise from observations of termination of atrial tachycardias originating from the LAA,[89,90] spontaneous conversion to sinus rhythm in cohort of patients with persistent or longstanding persistent AF who underwent LAA ligation for prevention of LAA thrombus formation,[91] and a decrease in AF burden in patients with cardiac implantable electronic devices who underwent successful LAA exclusion.[92] LAA ligation produces a debulking of the LA with significant beneficial electrical remodeling.[60–62] LAA ligation with PVI resulted in a significant decrease in P-wave duration and P-wave dispersion, and this favorable LA remodeling was associated with maintenance of sinus rhythm.[61] The LAALA AF registry, a prospective, multicenter propensity-matched study, assessed the impact of adding the LAA epicardial exclusion procedure to conventional PVI in patients with persistent AF.[62] LAA ligation with PVI resulted in a significant reduction of recurrence of AF compared with PVI alone.

The aMAZE trial is a prospective, multicenter, randomized controlled study investigating (ClinicalTrials.gov, registration no. NCT02513797)[55] whether PVI plus LAA ligation will lead to increased efficacy in maintaining sinus rhythm in patients with persistent and long-standing persistent AF as compared with PVI only (ClinicalTrials.gov, registration no. NCT02513797).[93] The trial consisted of randomizing 600 patients in a 2:1 randomization of PVI plus LAA ligation to PVI only. The primary end points include freedom from documented AF and other atrial arrhythmias of more than 30 seconds at 12 months after the PVI off antiarrhythmic drugs and 30-day safety of the LARIAT procedure. The composite of cardiovascular death and stroke as well as quality of life is a notable secondary outcome. The trial completed enrollment in December 2019 with 12-month follow-up data completed in April 2021. Results of the trial are expected to be known late 2021.

Ancillary benefit to epicardial LAA exclusion for LAA electrical isolation allows for a more extensive ablation of the left lateral ridge and LAA os without concern for LAA perforation, thrombus formation, and high recurrence rates seen with LAA electrical isolation with catheter ablation.[87,94,95] Atrial tachycardia foci originating from the LAA os and epicardial structures as the ligament of Marshall and autonomic ganglia plexi with its medial extensions into the left lateral ridge may be disrupted with endocardial ablation of the LAA os and lateral ridge owing to the less than 3 mm proximity to the endocardial surface of the ligament of Marshall.[96–99] Interruption of the ligament of Marshall and autonomic nerve bundles improves AF ablation outcomes.[100]

## Homeostasis Effects

The LAA is a neuroendocrine organ and the major source of atrial natriuretic peptide (ANP). ANP concentration is 40 times higher in the LAA than in the rest of the atrial free wall and in the ventricles and regulates natriuresis and diuresis in response to volume expansion.[101] The main physiologic function of ANP is to reduce blood volume via its effect to increase renal sodium and water excretion.[102] ANP also affects vascular tone by direct vasodilatation and inhibition of renin secretion resulting in reduced production of angiotensin and aldosterone.[103] This neuroendocrine response to LAA dilatation causes a decrease in blood volume, blood pressure, and serum sodium resulting in improved cardiac function.

Epicardial closure of the LAA is associated with an acute decrease in ANP levels in the first 24 hours after epicardial LAA closure that normalizes by 3 months.[104,105] In addition, the adrenergic neurohormones, adrenaline and noradrenaline, aldosterone, and renin, were found to be reduced for at least 3 months. The reduction of the adrenergic neurohormones and right atrium system also led to a decrease in blood pressure seen with both the AtriClip device and the LARIAT epicardial exclusion that is not observed with LAA endocardial occlusion.[104,106,107]

## Concerns with Epicardial Left Atrial Appendage Exclusion

Stand-alone LAA epicardial exclusion is currently performed with a left-sided thorascopic approach for the AtriClip device and an epicardial/endocardial percutaneous approach with the LARIAT suture delivery device. Either procedure is viewed as more complicated than catheter-based endocardial LAA occlusion devices. General anesthesia is required for both procedures. Deployment of the AtriClip device requires single-lung ventilation to allow for entering the pleural space, which some patients may not tolerate. The LARIAT procedure requires a "dry" pericardiocentesis that increases the risks of cardiac injury. However, with adequate training, both procedures can be performed with acceptable adverse event rates. Both procedures need pericardial drainage, thus generally requiring initial intensive care unit observation. Hospital stays are 2 to 3 days. Owing to producing ischemic necrosis of the LAA, a profound inflammatory response may occur, which has been associated with delayed pericardial effusions with the LARIAT or pleural effusions with the AtriClip device.[53,71] The postinflammatory pericardial effusions have been mitigated with vigilant pericardial drainage, pretreatment with colchicine, use of nonsteroidal anti-inflammatory drugs. In addition, early diagnosis of delayed pericardial effusions with a transthoracic echocardiogram 1 to 2 weeks postprocedure further allows for the management of delayed pericardial effusions.

Epicardial LAA exclusion leads to an acute release of ANP and affects the renin-angiotensin-aldosterone system and sympathetic neurohormes.[104,105] In rare cases, severe hypotension and hyponatremia can occur immediately after epicardial exclusion requiring pressor support and hypertonic saline. The hypotension and hyponatremia generally resolve within 24 to 48 hours. Between 24 hours and 3 months, LAA exclusion eliminates ANP release and blunts renal excretion of sodium and water after a large acute volume load.[108,109] In these circumstances, patients may experience fluid overload and require diuretics. However, the recent ATLAS and LAAOS III trials did not report an increased incidence of CHF hospitalizations.[81,82]

Because the LARIAT suture is deployed epicardially, patients with prior open-heart surgery and history of pericardial adhesions are contraindicated. Pectus excavatum and morbid obesity are also relative contraindications to the LARIAT procedure. In addition, because the approach to the LAA of the LARIAT suture delivery device is from anterior to posterior (surface of RV to the posteriorly located LAA), LAA morphologies in which the tip of the LAA is posterior to the pulmonary artery, a superior oriented LAA in which the tip is directed posteriorly, and an LAA width greater than 50 mm are also contraindications to the LARIAT procedure. The LAA morphologic restrictions for the LARIAT are barriers for the AtriClip device.

## Disclosure

RJL is a part-time Medical Director of AtriCure. TH is a consultant to AtriCure.

## CLINICS CARE POINTS

- Surgical LAA exclusion during a concomitant procedure should be considered in all patients with AF.
- Care must be taken to eliminate all LAA lobes and trabeculated LAA tissue.
- TEE guidance during stand-alone epicardial LAA exclusion should be used to assure that all LAA lobes are eliminated and there is no excessive remnant neck/stump.
- Extreme diligence during endocardial suture ligation of the LAA must be taken since the closure result can only be assessed after the heart is re-perfused, after the opportunity to rectify incomplete closure has passed.
- Epicardial LAA exclusion with the AtriClip or LARIAT produces ischemic necrosis of the LAA, a profound inflammatory response may occur which has been associated with delayed pericardial and/or pleural effusions. These are mitigated with the use of anti-inflamatory agents as NSAIDs, colchicine or steroids.
- Epicardial LAA exclusion leads to an acute release of ANP; and in rare cases, severe hypotension and hyponatremia can occur immediately after epicardial exclusion requiring pressor support and hypertonic saline. The hypotension and hyponatremia generally resolve within 24 to 48 hours.

## SUMMARY

LAA epicardial exclusion has been associated with addressing 2 potential deleterious consequences attributed to the LAA, namely, thrombus formation and an arrhythmogenic contributor, in advanced forms of AF. In addition, recent data suggest that modulation of the neuroendocrine effects of the LAA may beneficially lead to hypertension control. The recent results of the LAAOS III and ATLAS trials provide evidence that epicardial exclusion of the LAA should be considered with open-heart surgery. Future results of the aMAZE trial will provide information of the benefits of LAA electrical isolation using the LARIAT LAA exclusion system with catheter PVI ablation for persistent and longstanding persistent AF.

## REFERENCES

1. Go AS, Hylek EM, Phillips KA, et al. Prevalence of diagnosed atrial fibrillation in adults: national implications for rhythm management and stroke prevention: the Anticoagulation and Risk Factors

in Atrial Fibrillation (ATRIA) Study. JAMA 2001; 285(18):2370–5.

2. January CT, Wann LS, Alpert JS, et al. 2014 AHA/ ACC/HRS guideline for the management of patients with atrial fibrillation: a report of the American College of Cardiology/American Heart Association Task Force on Practice Guidelines and the Heart Rhythm Society. Circulation 2014; 130:2071–104.

3. Di Biase L, Burkhardt JD, Mohanty P, et al. Left atrial appendage: an underrecognized trigger site of atrial fibrillation. Circulation 2010;122(2):109–18.

4. Sanchez-Quintana D, Lopez-Minguez JR, Macias Y, et al. Left atrial anatomy relevant to catheter ablation. Cardiol Res Pract 2014;2014: 289720.

5. Blackshear JL, Odell JA. Appendage obliteration to reduce stroke in cardiac surgical patients with atrial fibrillation. Ann Thorac Surg 1996;61(2):755–9.

6. Lip GY, Tse HF. Management of atrial fibrillation. Lancet 2007;370(9587):604–18.

7. Wolf PA, Abbott RD, Kannel WB. Atrial fibrillation as an independent risk factor for stroke: the Framingham Study. Stroke 1991;22(8):983–8.

8. Hart RG, Halperin JL. Atrial fibrillation and stroke: concepts and controversies. Stroke 2001;32(3): 803–8.

9. Rosamond W, Flegal K, Furie K, et al. Heart disease and stroke statistics–2008 update: a report from the American Heart Association Statistics Committee and Stroke Statistics Subcommittee. Circulation 2008;117(4):e25–146.

10. Assiri A, Al-Majzoub O, Kanaan AO, et al. Mixed treatment comparison meta-analysis of aspirin, warfarin, and new anticoagulants for stroke prevention in patients with nonvalvular atrial fibrillation. Clin Ther 2013;35(7):967–984 e962.

11. Cruz-Flores S. Alternatives to long-term anticoagulation. Medscape 2014. Available at: http:// emedicine.medscape.com/article/1160021-overview#aw2aab6b7. Accessed July 14, 2014.

12. Fuster V, Rydén LE, Cannom DS, et al. ACC/AHA/ ESC 2006 guidelines for the management of patients with atrial fibrillation: full text: a report of the American College of Cardiology/American Heart Association Task Force on practice guidelines and the European Society of Cardiology Committee for Practice Guidelines (writing committee to revise the 2001 guidelines for the management of patients with atrial fibrillation) developed in collaboration with the European Heart Rhythm Association and the Heart Rhythm Society. Europace 2006;8(9):651–745.

13. Onalan O, Crystal E. Left atrial appendage exclusion for stroke prevention in patients with non-rheumatic atrial fibrillation. Stroke 2007;38(2): 624–30.

14. Kannel WB, Benjamin EJ. Status of the epidemiology of atrial fibrillation. Med Clin North America 2008;92(1):17–40, ix.

15. Lloyd-Jones D, Adams R, Carnethon M, et al. Heart disease and stroke statistics–2009 update: a report from the American Heart Association Statistics Committee and Stroke Statistics Subcommittee. Circulation 2009;119(3):480–6.

16. Blackshear JL, Johnson WD, Odell JA, et al. Thoracoscopic extracardiac obliteration of the left atrial appendage for stroke risk reduction in atrial fibrillation. J Am Coll Cardiol 2003;42(7):1249–52.

17. Haïssaguerre M, Jaïs P, Shah DC, et al. Spontaneous initiation of atrial fibrillation by ectopic beats originating in the pulmonary veins. N Engl J Med 1998;339(10):659–66.

18. Al-Saady NM, Obel OA, Camm AJ. Left atrial appendage: structure, function, and role in thromboembolism. Heart 1999;82(5):547–54.

19. Healey JS, Crystal E, Lamy A, et al. Left Atrial Appendage Occlusion Study (LAAOS): results of a randomized controlled pilot study of left atrial appendage occlusion during coronary bypass surgery in patients at risk for stroke. Am Heart J 2005; 150(2):288–93.

20. Beal JM, William P, Longmire J, et al. Resection of the auricular appendages. Ann Surg 1950;132(3):517–27.

21. Belcher JR, Somerville W. Systemic embolism and left auricular thrombosis in relation to mitral valvotomy. Br Med J 1955;4946(2):1000–3.

22. Cox JL. The surgical treatment of atrial fibrillation: IV. Surgical technique. J Thorac Cardiovasc Surg 1991;101:584–92.

23. Jordan R, Scheifley C, edwards J. Mural thrombosis and arterial embolism in mitral stenosis; a clinico-pathologic study of fifty-one cases. Circulation 1951;3(3):363–7.

24. American College of C. American Heart Association Task Force on Practice G, Society of Cardiovascular A, et al. ACC/AHA 2006 guidelines for the management of patients with valvular heart disease: a report of the American College of Cardiology/American Heart Association Task Force on Practice Guidelines (writing Committee to Revise the 1998 guidelines for the management of patients with valvular heart disease) developed in collaboration with the Society of Cardiovascular Anesthesiologists endorsed by the Society for Cardiovascular Angiography and Interventions and the Society of Thoracic Surgeons. J Am Coll Cardiol 2006;48(3):e1–148.

25. European Heart Rhythm A, Heart Rhythm S, Fuster V, et al. ACC/AHA/ESC 2006 guidelines for the management of patients with atrial fibrillation–executive summary: a report of the American College of Cardiology/American Heart Association Task Force on Practice Guidelines and the

European Society of Cardiology Committee for Practice Guidelines (writing committee to revise the 2001 guidelines for the management of patients with atrial fibrillation). J Am Coll Cardiol 2006;48(4):854–906.

26. American Heart Association ACoCF. ACCF/AHA pocket guideline: management of patients with atrial fibrillation. Elsevier. 2011. Available at: http://www.cardiosource.org/~/media/Files/Science%20and%20Quality/Guidelines/Pocket%20Guides/AFIB_PocketGuide.ashx. Accessed July 13, 2011.

27. Camm AJ, Lip GYH, De Caterina R, et al. 2012 Focused update of the ESC guidelines for the management of atrial fibrillation: an update of the 2010 ESC Guidelines for the management of atrial fibrillation developed with the special contribution of the European Heart Rhythm Association. Europace 2012;14(10):1385–413.

28. NIfHaC Excellence. Atrial fibrillation: the management of atrial fibrillation. CG180 Web site. 2014. Available at: http://www.nice.org.uk/guidance/cg180/resources/guidance-atrial-fibrillation-the-management-of-atrial-fibrillation-pdf. Updated November 2014. Accessed.

29. Johnson WD, Ganjoo AK, Stone CD, et al. The left atrial appendage: our most lethal human attachment! Surgical implications. Eur J cardiothoracic Surg 2000;17(6):718–22.

30. García-Fernández Mn, Pérez-David E, Quiles J, et al. Role of left atrial appendage obliteration in stroke reduction in patients with mitral valve prosthesis: a transesophageal echocardiographic study. J Am Coll Cardiol 2003;42(7):1253–8.

31. Apostolakis E, Papakonstantinou NA, Baikoussis NG, et al. Surgical strategies and devices for surgical exclusion of the left atrial appendage: a word of caution. J Cardiovasc Surg 2013;28(2):199–206.

32. Fisher DC, Tunick PA, Kronzon I. Large gradient across a partially ligated left atrial appendage. J Am Soc Echocardiogr 1998;11:1163.

33. Katz ES, Tsiamtsiouris T, Applebaum RM, et al. Surgical left atrial appendage ligation is frequently incomplete: a transesophageal echocardiograhic study. J Am Coll Cardiol 2000;36:468–71.

34. Rosenzweig BP, Katz E, Kort S, et al. Thromboembolus from a ligated left atrial appendage. J Am Soc Echocardiogr 2001;14:396–8.

35. DiSesa VJ, Tam S, Cohn LH. Ligation of the left atrial appendage using an automatic surgical stapler. Ann Thorac Surg 1988;46:652–3.

36. Kanderian AS, Gillinov AM, Pettersson GB, et al. Success of surgical left atrial appendage closure: assessment by transesophageal echocardiography. J Am Coll Cardiol 2008;52:924–9.

37. Gillinov AM, Pettersson G Cosgrove DM. Stapled excision of the left atrial appendage. J Thorac Cardiovasc Surg 2005;129:679–80.

38. Bakhtiary F, Kleine P, Martens S, et al. Simplified technique for surgical ligation of the left atrial appendage in high-risk patients. J Thorac Cardiovasc Surg 2008;135:430–1.

39. Damiano RJ Jr, Gaynor SL, Bailey M, et al. The long-term outcome of patients with coronary disease and atrial fibrillation undergoing the Cox maze procedure. J Thorac Cardiovasc Surg 2003;126(6):2016–21.

40. Kamohara K, Fukamachi K, Ootaki Y, et al. A novel device for left atrial appendage exclusion. J Thorac Cardiovasc Surg 2005;130(6):1639–44.

41. Kamohara K, Fukamachi K, Ootaki Y, et al. Evaluation of a novel device for left atrial appendage exclusion: the second-generation atrial exclusion device. J Thorac Cardiovasc Surg 2006;132(2):340–6.

42. Fumoto H, Gillinov AM, Ootaki Y, et al. A novel device for left atrial appendage exclusion: the third-generation atrial exclusion device. J Thorac Cardiovasc Surg 2008;136(4):1019–27.

43. Salzberg SP, Plass A, Emmert MY, et al. Left atrial appendage clip occlusion: early clinical results. J Thorac Cardiovasc Surg 2010;139(5):1269–74.

44. Ailawadi G, Gerdisch MW, Harvey RL, et al. Exclusion of the left atrial appendage with a novel device: early results of a multicenter trial. J Thorac Cardiovasc Surg 2011;142(5):1002–9.e1001.

45. Emmert MY, Puippe G, Baumuller S, et al. Safe, effective and durable epicardial left atrial appendage clip occlusion in patients with atrial fibrillation undergoing cardiac surgery: first long-term results from a prospective device trial. Eur J cardio-thoracic Surg 2014;45(1):126–31.

46. Ad N, Massimiano PS, Shuman DJ, et al. New approach to exclude the left atrial appendage during minimally invasive Cryothermic surgical ablation. Innovations (Phila) 2015;10(5):323–7.

47. Alqaqa A, Martin S, Hamdan A, et al. Concomitant left atrial appendage clipping during minimally invasive mitral valve surgery: technically feasible and safe. J Atr Fibrillation 1941;9:1407–6911.

48. Page S, Hallam J, Pradhan N, et al. Left atrial appendage exclusion using the AtriClip device: a case series. Heart Lung Circ 2019;28(3):430–5.

49. Caliskan E, Eberhard M, Falk V, et al. Incidence and characteristics of left atrial appendage stumps after device-enabled epicardial closure. Interact Cardiovasc Thorac Surg 2019;29(5):663–9.

50. Yoshimoto A, Suematsu Y, Kurahashi K, et al. Early and middle-term results and anticoagulation strategy after left atrial appendage exclusion using an epicardial clip device. Ann Thorac Cardiovasc Surg 2020;27(3):185–90.

51. Ellis CR, Aznaurov SG, Patel NJ, et al. Angiographic efficacy of the AtriClip left atrial appendage exclusion device placed by minimally invasive thorascopic approach. JACC Clin Electrophysiol 2017;3(12):1356–65.

52. Toale C, Fitzmaurice GJ, Eaton D, et al. Outcomes of left atrial appendage occlusion using the AtriClip device: a systematic review. Interact Cardiovasc Thorac Surg 2019;29(5):655–62.

53. Bartus K, Han FT, Bednarek J, et al. Percutaneous left atrial appendage suture ligation using the LARIAT device in patients with atrial fibrillation: initial clinical experience. J Am Coll Cardiol 2013;62(2):108–18.

54. Koneru JN, Badhwar N, Ellenbogen KA, et al. LAA ligation using the LARIAT suture delivery device: tips and tricks for a successful procedure. Heart Rhythm 2014;11:911–21.

55. Lee RJ, Bartus K, Yakubov SJ. Catheter-based left atrial appendage (LAA) ligation for the prevention of embolic events arising from the LAA: initial experience in a canine model. Circ Cardiovasc Interv 2010;3(3):224–9.

56. Bartus K, Morelli RL, Szczepanski W, et al. Anatomic analysis of the left atrial appendage after closure with the LARIAT device. Circ Arrhythm Electrophysiol 2014;7(4):764–7.

57. Ellis CR, Byrd JM, Scalf SL. Ischemic necrosis of the left atrial appendage at autopsy 4 weeks following epicardial suture ligation via a subxiphoid approach (LARIAT). J Interv Card Electrophysiol 2015;43(1):99–100.

58. Sievert H, Rasekh A, Bartus K, et al. Left atrial appendage ligation in nonvalvular atrial fibrillation patients at high risk for embolic events with ineligibility for oral anticoagulation: initial report of clinical outcomes. JACC Clin Electrophysiol 2015;1(6):465–74.

59. Han FT, Bartus K, Lakkireddy D, et al. The effects of LAA ligation on LAA electrical activity. Heart Rhythm 2014;11(5):864–70.

60. Kawamura M, Scheinman MM, Lee RJ, et al. Left atrial appendage ligation in patients with atrial fibrillation leads to a decrease in atrial dispersion. J Am Heart Assoc 2015;4(5).

61. Badhwar N, Lakkireddy D, Kawamura M, et al. Sequential percutaneous LAA ligation and pulmonary vein isolation in patients with persistent AF: initial results of a feasibility study. J Cardiovasc Electrophysiol 2015;26(6):608–14.

62. Lakkireddy D, Mahankali AS, Kanmanthareddy A, et al. Left atrial appendage ligation and ablation for persistent atrial fibrillation (LAALA-AF registry). J Am Coll Cardiol EP 2015;1:153–60.

63. Bartus K, Bednarek J, Myc J, et al. Feasibility of closed-chest ligation of the left atrial appendage in humans. Heart Rhythm 2011;8(2):188–93.

64. Bartus K, Gafoor S, Tschopp D, et al. Left atrial appendage ligation with the next generation LARIAT(+) suture delivery device: early clinical experience. Int J Cardiol 2016;215:244–7.

65. Sanchez JM, Lee A, Bartus K, et al. Percutaneous epicardial approach for LAA ligation. J Interv Card Electrophysiol 2020. https://doi.org/10.1007/s10840-020-00894-9.

66. Massumi A, Chelu MG, Nazeri A, et al. Initial experience with a novel percutaneous left atrial appendage exclusion device in patients with atrial fibrillation, increased stroke risk, and contraindications to anticoagulation. Am J Cardiol 2013;111:869–73.

67. Stone D, Byrne T, Pershad A. Early results with the LARIAT device for left atrial appendage exclusion in patients with atrial fibrillation at high risk for stroke and anticoagulation. Catheter Cardiovasc Interv 2013. https://doi.org/10.1002/ccd.25065.

68. Price MJ, Gibson DN, Yakubov SJ, et al. Early safety and efficacy of percutaneous left atrial appendage suture ligation: results from the U.S. transcatheter LAA ligation consortium. J Am Coll Cardiol 2014;64:565–72.

69. Miller MA, Gangireddy SR, Doshi SK, et al. Multicenter study on acute and long-term safety and efficacy of percutaneous left atrial appendage closure using an epicardial suture snaring device. Heart Rhythm 2014;11:1853–9.

70. Gunda S, Reddy M, Pillarisetti J, et al. Differences in complication rates between large bore needle and a long micropuncture needle during epicardial access: time to change clinical practice? Circ Arrhythm Electrophysiol 2015;8:890–5.

71. Lakkireddy D, Afzal MR, Lee RJ, et al. Short and long-term outcomes of percutaneous left atrial appendage suture ligation: results from a US multicenter evaluation. Heart Rhythm 2016;13(5):1030–6.

72. Tilz RR, Fink T, Bartus K, et al. A collective European experience with left atrial appendage suture ligation using the LARIAT+ device. Europace 2020;22(6):924–31.

73. Yamamoto M, Seo Y, Kawamatsu N, et al. Complex left atrial appendage morphology and left atrial appendage thrombus formation in patients with atrial fibrillation. Circ Cardiovasc Imaging 2014;7:337–43.

74. Undas A, Zabczyk M. Plasma fibrin clot structure and thromboembolism: clinical implications. Pol Arch Intern Med 2017;127(12):873–81.

75. Roldan V, Marin F, Biann A, et al. Interleukin-6, endothelial activation and thrombogenesis in chronic atrial fibrillation. Eur Heart J 2003;24(14):1373–80.

76. Sadanaga T, Kohsaka S, Ogawa S. D-dimer levels in combination with clinical risk factors can

effectively predict subsequent thromboembolic events in patients with atrial fibrillation during oral anticoagulant therapy. Cardiology 2010; 117(1):31–6.

77. Bartus K, Podolec J, Lee RJ, et al. Atrial natriuretic peptide and brain natriuretic peptide changes after epicardial percutaneous left atrial appendage suture ligation using LARIAT device. J Physiol And Pharmacol 2017;68(1):117–23.

78. Cox JL, Ad N, Palazzo T. Impact of the maze procedure on the stroke rate in patients with atrial fibrillation. J Thorac Cardiovasc Surg 1999;118(5):833–40.

79. Madden JL. Resection of the left auricular appendix; a prophylaxis for recurrent arterial emboli. J Am Med Assoc 1949;140(9):769–72.

80. Caliskan Etem, Sahin Ayhan, Yilmaz Murat, Seifert Burkhardt, Hinzpeter Ricarda, Alkadhi Hatem, Cox James L, Holubec Tomas, Reser Diana, Falk Volkmar, Grünenfelder Jürg, Genoni Michele, Maisano Francesco, Salzberg Sacha P, Emmert Maximilian Y. Epicardial left atrial appendage AtriClip occlusion reduces the incidence of stroke in patients with atrial fibrillation undergoing cardiac surgery. Europace (London, England) 2018;20(7):e105–14.

81. Gerdisch MW, Edward Garrett H, Mumtaz MA, et al. Prophylactic left atrial appendance exclusion in patients undergoing cardiac surgery: results of the prospective, multi-center, randomized ATLAS trial. Boston, MA: Presented at Heart Rhythm Society; 2021.

82. Whitlock RP, Belley-Cote EP, Paparella D, et al. for the LAAOS III Investigators. Left atrial appendage occlusion during cardiac surgery to prevent. stroke. N Engl J Med 2021;384:2081–91.

83. Olshansky B, Heller EN, Mitchell LB, et al. Are transthoracic echocardiographic parameters associated with atrial fibrillation recurrence or stroke? Results from the Atrial Fibrillation Follow-Up Investigation of Rhythm Management (AFFIRM) study. J Am Coll Cardiol 2005;45(12):2026–33. https://doi.org/10.1016/j.jacc.2005.03.020.

84. Njoku A, Kannabhiran M, Arora R, et al. Left atrial volume predicts atrial fibrillation recurrence after radiofrequency ablation: a meta-analysis. Europace 2018;20(1):33–42.

85. Masahiro ogawa MD, Koichiro kumagai MD, Marta vakulenko MD, et al. Reduction of P-wave duration and successful pulmonary vein isolation in patients with atrial fibrillation. J Chem Ecol 2007;18:931–8.

86. Katarina Van Beeumen, Houben Richard, Tavernier Rene, et al. Changes in P-wave area and P-wave duration after circumferential pulmonary vein isolation. Europace 2010;12(6):798–804.

87. Fink T, Schlüter M, Heeger CH, et al. Combination of left atrial appendage isolation and ligation to treat nonresponders of pulmonary vein isolation. JACC Clin Electrophysiol 2018;4(12):1569–79.

88. Starck C, Steffel J, Emmert MY, et al. Epicardial left atrial appendage clip occlusion also provides the electrical isolation of the left atrial appendage. Interactive CardioVascular Thorac Surg 2012;15:416–9.

89. Atoui M, Pillarisetti J, Iskandar S, et al. Left atrial appendage tachycardia termination with a LARIAT suture ligation. J Atr Fibrillation 2015;8(4):1380.

90. Benussi S, Mazzone P, Maccabelli G, et al. Thoracoscopic appendage exclusion with an AtriClip device as a solo treatment for focal atrial tachycardia. Circulation 2011;123(14):1575–8.

91. Badhwar N, Mittal S, Rasekh A, et al. Conversion of persistent atrial fibrillation to sinus rhythm after LAA ligation with the LARIAT device. Int J Cardiol 2016;225:120–2.

92. Afzal MR, Kanmanthareddy A, Earnest M, et al. Impact of left atrial appendage exclusion using an epicardial ligation system (LARIAT) on atrial fibrillation burden in patients with cardiac implantable electronic devices. Heart Rhythm 2015;12(1):52–9.

93. Lee RJ, Lakkireddy D, Mittal S, et al. Percutaneous alternative to the Maze procedure for the treatment of persistent or long-standing persistent atrial fibrillation (aMAZE trial): rationale and design. Am Heart J 2015;170(6):1184–94.

94. Di Biase L, Burkhardt JD, Mohanty P, et al. Left atrial appendage isolation in patients with long-standing persistent AF undergoing catheter ablation. J Am Coll Cardiol 2016;68:1929–40.

95. Rillig A, Tilz RR, Lin T, et al. Unexpectedly high incidence of stroke and left atrial appendage thrombus formation after electrical isolation of the left atrial appendage for the treatment of atrial tachyarrhythmias. Circ Arrhythnmia Electrophysiol 2016;9(5):e003461.

96. Chik WW, Chan JK, Ross DL, et al. Atrial tachycardias utilizing the ligament of Marshall region following single ring pulmonary vein isolation for atrial fibrillation. Pacing Clin Electrophysiol 2014; 37:1149–58.

97. Kim DT, Lai AC, Hwang C, et al. The ligament of Marshall: a structural analysis in human hearts with implications for atrial arrhythmias. J Am Coll Cardiol 2000;36:1324–7.

98. Cabrera JA, Ho SY, Climent V, et al. The architecture of the left lateral atrial wall: a particular anatomic region with implications for ablation of atrial fibrillation. Eur Heart J 2008;29:356–62.

99. Hwang C, Fishbein MC, Chen PS. How and when to ablate the ligament of Marshall. Heart Rhythm 2006;3(12):1505–7.

100. Valderrabano M, Pederson LE, Swarup V, et al. Effect of catheter ablation with vein of Marshall

ethanol infusion vs catheter ablation alone on persistent atrial fibrillation the VENUS randomized clinical trial. JAMA 2020;324:1620–8.

101. Rodeheffer RJ, Naruse M, Atkinson JB, et al. Molecular forms of atrial natriuretic factor in normal and failing human myocardium. Circulation 1993; 88:364–71.

102. Theilig F, Wu Q. ANP-induced signaling cascade and its implications in renal pathophysiology. Am J Phys Renal Phys 2015;308(10):F1047–55.

103. Nishikimi T, Maeda N, Matsuoka H. The role of natriuretic peptides in cardioprotection. Cardiovasc Res 2006;69:318–28.

104. Lakkireddy D, Turagam M, Afzal MR, et al. Left atrial appendage closure and systemic homeostasis: the LAA HOMEOSTASIS study. J Am Coll Cardiol 2018;71:135–44.

105. Bartus K, Podolec J, Lee RJ, et al. Atrial natriuretic peptide and brain natriuretic peptide changes after epicardial percutaneous left atrial appendage suture ligation using LARIAT device. J Physiol Pharmacol 2017;68:117–23.

106. Maybrook R, Pillarisetti J, Yarlagadda V, et al. Electrolyte and hemodynamic changes following percutaneous left atrial appendage ligation with the LARIAT device. J Interv Card Electrophysiol 2015;43:245–51.

107. Turagam MK, Vuddanda V, Verberkmoes N, et al. Epicardial left atrial appendage exclusion reduces blood pressure in patients with atrial fibrillation and hypertension. J Am Coll Cardiol 2018;72(12):1346–53.

108. Stewart JM, Dean R, Brown M, et al. Bilateral atrial appendectomy abolishes increased plasma atrial natriuretic peptide release and blunts sodium and water excretion during volume loading in conscious dogs. Circ Res 1992;70:724–32.

109. Omari BO, Nelson RJ, Robertson JM. Effect of right atrial appendectomy on the release of atrial natriuretic hormone. J Thorac Cardiovasc Surg 1991;102:272–9.

# The Future of LAAC—In 5, 10, and 20 Years

Matthew J. Daniels, BSc, MA, MB, BChir, PhD, MRCP, FSCAI[a,b,c,*],
Adrian Parry-Jones, MD[b,d,e]

## KEYWORDS

- Left atrial appendage • Device thrombus • Invasive pressure monitor • Atrial fibrillation
- Oral anticoagulant • Intracerebral hemorrhage

## KEY POINTS

- LAA closure is an emerging field, this article considers the future directions it may take over the next 5, 10, and 20 years.
- To change routine practice a superior trial outcome over direct oral anticoagulants is needed.
- The health economic arguments for LAA closure will change as direct oral anticoagulant patents expire (due 2023–27).
- Additional health economic impacts may be realized if implantable monitoring capabilities relevant to heart failure can be incorporated into LAAC devices.
- Improvements in procedure safety and efficacy will continue to accrue through multiple discrete improvements in patient selection, device development, and postprocedure management.

## INTRODUCTION

It is always dangerous to predict the future, but if the point of this series of articles is to cover the current state of the field of LAAC—warts and all—it seems reasonable to offer a road map of the major transitions we can expect, and the timelines they may occur over. MJD is currently influenced by the series of predictions made on an annual basis by @pknoepfler on Twitter[1] on another rapidly moving field in biology and medicine (cell therapy). They are not always right, but also not always wrong. By committing to a position you can learn more about how a field is evolving more meaningfully than when a passive observer role is taken. Here we similarly try to construct an article based on predictions, with associated justifications, over the next few pages on LAAC. Paradoxically we believe it will be easier to predict whereby we will be in 20 years compared with any intermediary time point so we start in +20 years, when we are both due to be retiring, and possibly looking for someone to close our LAA.

## PREDICTION 1: WHERE LAAC WILL BE IN 20 YEARS?

People who don't learn from history are doomed to repeat it. If that is the case you

Tweet: Predictions for the future of LAAC – a simple path to success?

Conflicts: M.J. Daniels research grant & speaker honorarium Abbott, Consultant – WL GORE & Associates, Advisory Board fees Bristol Myers Squibb; A. Parry-Jones Speaker and Advisory Board fees from Alexion Pharmaceuticals.

[a] Manchester Heart Centre, Manchester Royal Infirmary, Manchester University NHS Foundation Trust, UK; [b] Division of Cardiovascular Sciences, Manchester Academic Health Sciences Centre, University of Manchester, UK; [c] Division of Cell Matrix Biology and Regenerative Medicine, University of Manchester, Manchester, UK; [d] Geoffrey Jefferson Brain Research Centre, Manchester Academic Health Science Centre, Northern Care Alliance & University of Manchester, Manchester UK; [e] Manchester Centre for Clinical Neurosciences, Northern Care Alliance NHS Group, Stott Lane, Salford M6 8HD, UK

* Corresponding author. Institute of Cardiovascular Sciences, Core Technology Facility, University of Manchester, Room 3.20, 46 Grafton Street, Manchester M13 9NT, United Kingdom.

*E-mail address:* matthew.daniels@manchester.ac.uk

Twitter: @cardiacpolymath (M.J.D.)

2211-7458/22/© 2021 Elsevier Inc. All rights reserved.

| Abbreviations | |
|---|---|
| DOAC | Direct Oral Anti-Coagulant |
| ICH | Intracerebral hemorrhage |
| LAA | Left Atrial Appendage |
| LAAC | Left Atrial Appendage Closure |
| PFO | Patent Foramen Ovale |
| TAVI | Transcatheter Aortic Valve Implantation |

could argue that the interval from the first surgical amputation of the LAA in the 1940's—in dogs[2] and humans[3] to the recent announcement of the LAAOSIII results[4] suggests that in 20 years LAAC will be no further on than it is at present. After all, the skill of the cardiac surgeon combined with the established technologies of stainless steel and surgical silk can effectively pacify any appendage anatomy at virtually zero cost. If it takes the best part of a century to prove the utility of LAA excision surgically what are the chances for a device strategy in 20 years?

Naturally, cardiologists will wish to distance themselves from the slow progress of our surgical cousins—well at least the English ones will. So at this point, it is useful to pause, and reflect, that we are now celebrating the 20-year anniversary of the first device-based LAA closures[5,6] (which occurred in 2001). In the interval, we have effectively managed to coordinate and execute, one randomized study (PROTECTAF, PREVAIL[7,8]), for one device (Watchman), in less than 1000 patients. Are we really on a different trajectory than the surgeons?

We think we are, but that difference is driven by device industry involvement for development and manufacture. As they are now pivoting their considerable R&D efforts toward new markets like LAAC—and away from established markets (eg pacing and coronary stents) —their cumulative investment/exposure means that our timelines will now shorten. The recent, and rapid turn round in the Amulet IDE trial,[9] and the PINNACLE FLX[10] study attest to this, and give rise to the first prediction:

> In 20 years we will know if LAAc is futile (in which case it will be on the shelf of good ideas that didn't work out) or if it is prognostically useful (in which case it will be a routine, facile procedure, offered much earlier in life than we currently consider it). The LAAOSIII result pushes us towards the later outcome, and we are optimistic that many parallels to PFO closure will emerge

with ∼95% of patients being possible to treat with one approach, in a ∼30-minute day-case procedure with major complications less than 1/500 in most operators hands.

It is fair to note this is not much of a prediction—it will work, or it won't, so what makes us think we will iterate toward this positive outcome? What are the steps needed to get there?

## PREDICTION 2: TRIAL OUTCOMES AND IMPACTS

As others have observed[11] the trial landscape for LAAc is dominated by the availability of alternative therapies to reduce stroke typically recommended to patients with atrial fibrillation—the anticoagulants. It has already proven impossible to recruit large numbers of patients who are device eligible but DOAC ineligible into a trial environment exploring device/no device outcomes so the utility of LAAC in this cohort may never be answered definitively. This horse has bolted as guidelines already support closure in this patient group. Instead, extrapolation from the use of LAAC devices in DOAC eligible patient trials will be needed for this group of patients who at best will only have registry data.

Firstly, trials in the DOAC eligible will establish relevant procedure safety benchmarks. From this, we will be able to determine how much additional procedural risk the routinely treated DOAC ineligible group—which is generally older, sicker, and frailer—face. Paralleling the early transcatheter aortic valve implantation (TAVI) trials on surgically inoperable patients with severe aortic stenosis[12] which demonstrated the efficacy of a therapy in a patient population with a 6% 30d, and 30% 1-year mortality we can anticipate a similar "range finding" process to identify the equivalent "cohort C" of multiply comorbid patients who derive little from the risks of LAAC. Consequently, we will get better at not offering LAAC to patients who may have little to gain from the upfront procedure risk without the delayed benefits it promises. At present, the LAAC registry patients have a ∼10% annual mortality, suggesting that we have a long way to go.

Second, even if LAAC is proven noninferior to DOAC (in patients who can take it) it is not impossible to imagine that in national health care systems LAAC would remain restricted to the DOAC ineligible population on health economic grounds. Such decisions are based on the current pricing of medication, and procedure cost in the context of the age and life expectancy of the average patient. At present 10 years of DOAC *is cheaper than* LAAC with 10-year survival DOAC free. The expiry of DOAC drug patents would clearly be a disruptive event in this landscape—UK dates for this range from 2023 to 2027.

Third, *until a superiority result* is obtained in a randomized trial versus DOAC there will be minimal changes in clinical referral pathways or guidelines. Marginal gains to tilt the ice toward a successful device outcome will come from factors that improve procedure safety (peri-procedure imaging, sizing, alignment to reduce recapture and redeployment), and those that reduce early postimplant complications (reduce leak, device-related thrombus (DRT) formation, embolization). Concomitantly, the drug companies will be working on strategies that tilt the ice in the opposite direction developing safer anticoagulants. Finally, with the increasing availability of advanced medical imaging, and medically relevant information from consumer electronics (eg blood pressure, heart rate/rhythm), and even genetic information that might contribute to bleeding risk scores, it may become easier to identify subgroups at risk of bleeding for whom LAAC may be more useful—should trials in the all-comer population not reach superiority.

*We will have a definitive trial result in less than 10 years but might not get it right for first time. A superiority demonstration is needed to fundamentally change the landscape towards routine use. Health economic arguments will change rapidly as DOAC patents expire.*

## PREDICTION 3: A DOMINANT DEVICE STRATEGY

The natural history of all mature markets is that they come to be dominated by only a handful of providers. At present 2 dominant device concepts coexist, the plug,[13] and the lobe and disc.[14] For each category there is a clear "market leader" with the first mover advantage but many variations on these themes that have niche advantages.

Regarding efficacy, the only published real-world comparison[15] of the leading devices did not report a large difference in the real-world setting when it came to procedure success. These were broadly emulated in the string of noninferiority results covered in the recently published AMULET IDE study (for patients who had to have anatomy suitable for either device).[9] However, it is noted that this did identify a small, but significant, improvement in closure with the lobe and disc strategy, with fewer procedure failures, but with some increased risk of bleeding.

So, what about procedure-related harms like DRT[16]? Recent data on the location of thrombus following LAAC[17] suggest that the 2 strategies might not be equivalent—in theory at least. The AMULET IDE study actually found numerically less device thrombus overall in the patients treated by the lobe and disc device[9] which somewhat reverses the trend of prior literature. Furthermore, it is accepted that any intracardiac device may not be equivalent to surgical alternatives which leave no material behind.

We have observed that the LAA arising beneath the pulmonary vein (aka warfarin) ridge (which is variable in length and angulation) makes it possible to create a "neo-appendage" when the device tucks into the LAA (**Fig. 1**). This is a particular problem for the plug concept, but also a challenge for the lobe and disc devices when the warfarin ridge is long. It can be argued that such procedural outcomes have not closed the appendage they have simply made it smaller. Reducing the volume of the LAA may, or may not, impact on stroke risk. It may well be that a smaller anatomic site prevents the formation of large thrombi sufficiently protecting patients from large embolic strokes. However, the flow vortices in these cul-de-sacs do seem to allow thrombus formation,[18] and we now have clear data that show device thrombus is a risk of stroke following LAAC.[19,20]

Presently we lack data to confirm or refute the suggestion that one device strategy is better than another but it is possible to imagine that over a 10-year timeline we might see plug type devices evolve a disc (if this improves closure rates), or conversely lobe and disc devices losing the disc if this adds to procedure complexity without improving outcome.

All intracardiac devices may struggle to match the closure+ aspects of extracardiac LAA ligation which could impact intracardiac thrombus rates due to the lack of foreign body, and include LA remodeling, LAA electrical isolation, and putative homeostatic effects should these become established in extended analyses of reported or ongoing trial activity.[21]

*Within 10 years there will be a dominant strategy for LAAC—be that intracardiac or extracardiac.*

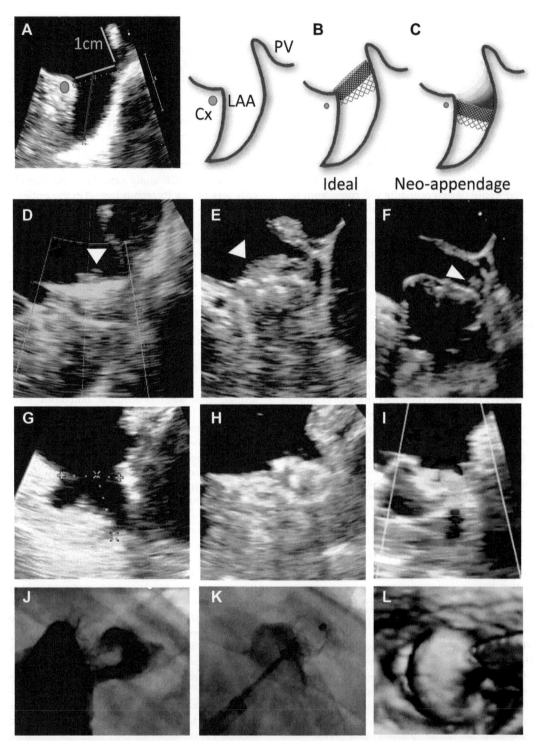

**Fig. 1.** The Neo-appendage concept: (*A*) A simple windsock LAA with standard markers for ostial sizing (*orange line*) and depth assessment (*red line*) at the level of the circumflex artery (*blue circle*). Note the warfarin (pulmonary vein) ridge projects ∼1 cm beyond the ostium (*green line*). The transesophageal echo on the left is stylized graphically on the right (Cx – Circumflex artery, PV – pulmonary vein). LAA devices deployed on the same arc may sit in an ideal position (*B*), or deeper in the LAA (*C*) reshaping the LAA rather than occluding it. This neo-appendage is a nidus for thrombus formation (*red*). Examples of DRT (*white arrow*) in simple LAA anatomy with neo-appendages created by warfarin ridges of different lengths: (*D*) small clot on an Amulet device; (*E*) dense clot

## PREDICTION 4: INCLUSION OF OTHER TECHNOLOGIES

At present, the medical device market looking for a home in the left atrium (or pulmonary arteries) resembles a student desk in the 1990s with a TV, video, stereo, PC, and printer competing for space. Now all these functions (and more) are combined into a smartphone that fits in a pocket.

The question for the LAAC devices is whether the current practice to obviate the structure is a missed opportunity to make use of the average volume of the left atrial appendage ($\sim$10 mL) for other purposes. The 2 most appealing technologies to incorporate relate to the overlap of atrial fibrillation and heart failure. Pulmonary artery pressure monitors have demonstrated utility in heart failure populations using a space-age technology that does not require a power source.[22] LA pressure monitoring is also possible,[23] and potentially more useful as most heart failure is a left ventricular problem. Knowing LA pressure independently of concomitant respiratory pathology may be an advantage. The ability to tailor diuretic therapy more closely in this patient group would be a clear route to reduce AF/heart failure hospitalizations. But can we imagine a device not just reporting high pressure (before heart failure symptoms develop) but also the report volume status heading too low (before orthostatic symptoms)? At the moment the focus is on numbers getting bigger, whereas numbers getting smaller are equally valuable because they can drive clinical events like falls which have health care costs also measured in $billions.

One of the advantages of the lobe and disc concept is such devices have a central spindle that is pulled into the LAA. It is not impossible to imagine that the degree of stretch in the connection, or curvature in the disc, may be possible to measure/transduce reporting on under-filling hence covering both ends of the pressure spectrum. Equally, just as LA pressure can be influenced by a preprocedure fast and require fluid administration to help device sizing, the daily fluctuations in filing may alter lobe compression in a way that may be possible to measure and convert into a hemodynamic signal relevant to heart failure.

A second technology to incorporate would be rate/rhythm and accelerometer data from implantable pacing technologies which have proven capability to discriminate activity by age, frailty, NYHA class, depravation index.[24] Rate or rhythm control strategies are an important aspect of managing patients with AF, and identifying better ways to select high-risk patients for ablation, or transitions to permanent pacing/ablation or medication titration based on objective data would be welcome.

If LAAC devices with these capabilities could be developed, without impacting on their implantation characteristics, it would seem to generate clear water between an intracardiac device (which could include monitoring) and the surgical exclusion (which would lack monitoring) approach.

The final relevant technology is some sort of device-related pharmacotherapy. This could address device thrombus in patients who are poor candidates for systemic antiplatelet or anticoagulant therapy. Although the natural assumption might be to engineer things with a "non-stick" coating, or even antiplatelet/coagulant eluting properties similar to the drug-eluting coronary stent[25] it might paradoxically not be unreasonable to go in completely the opposite direction and make devices that are proinflammatory (to generate scar) or even prothrombotic. This approach would almost certainly require concomitant use of OAC to prevent systemic sequela. However, by accelerating endothelialization in a patient group whereby this occurs slowly, and unpredictably, the aim would be to reach a definite end-point of complete scaring quickly rather than the current situation which is open-ended and often incomplete.

A similar concept may resolve another clinical conundrum. Currently, there is too much uncertainty in the assessment of device endothelialization. We struggle to tell whether this is complete

---

on top, and through, a Watchman device; (*F*) small clot at the distal end of a long neo-appendage created by a Watchman device. In more complex anatomy, for example, multilobe cactus LAA (*G*), the intent to plug the dominant lobe with a Watchman would always leave the proximal lobe uncovered (*H*). In this case, the device was released in the minor lobe leaving a large residual leak to the dominant lobe (*I, J*). This was large enough to accommodate a 12F Amulet delivery sheath, such that an Amulet lobe could be deployed behind the Watchman, and the disc used to cover the rest of the appendage (*K*). In (*L*), the 3D TOE image shows the disc retracted on the delivery cable revealing an arc of the initial Watchman 7 to 11 o'clock.

or not and cannot predict when it will be finished. Noninvasive imaging techniques will never have sufficient in vivo resolution to visualize this process as the thickness of an endocardial cell layer could be as little as ~20 µm. A biochemical marker—derived from the device, or a reaction to the device—might be easier to monitor. This could deliver a personalized postprocedure medication regimen based on the extent of coverage.

A completely different proposal might involve in vitro "cellularization" of devices before their implant using autologous cells, or those currently being engineered for general immuno-compatibility in the regenerative medicine context. Clearly, a barrier to these transitions will be the regulatory hurdles required of medicines; cell therapies are also classed as medicine in this regard. However, DRT is not uncommon (~5%) and is associated with stroke. It is a deeply uncomfortable diagnosis to make for both patient and treating physician in the context of guidelines positioning the treatment in those ineligible for the suite of treatments to resolve clot.[26] The clear association with stroke postprocedure[19,20] directly reduces the effectiveness of the therapy. Thus, although the clinical impact of this problem might be considered relatively minor, as most DRT is not linked to subsequent stroke, it is a problem worth paying attention to. By way of a parallel, can you imagine that PFO and ASD devices would be as broadly accepted if they had a 5% thrombus rate???

*In 10 years' time, LAAC devices will also be a barometer of the left atrium and cardiovascular health.*

## PREDICATION 5: REPOSITIONING LAAC TO YOUNGER PATIENTS

There seem to be certainties in the natural history of AF that current LAAC practice ignores. Once AF is identified it is likely to come back, and last longer, until it becomes permanent.[27] The stroke risk is not clearly linked to the AF burden—having a bit is just as bad as having a lot of it. Indeed, although successful cardioversion may reprogram the rhythm, it does not seem to reprogram the stroke risk.[28] Effectively once the atrium declares AF it declares an elevated stroke risk that persists lifelong.

This stroke risk is not static, it increases with age.

Age also plays into interventional cardiology in a couple of ways—complications, and healing.

Major complications occur during LAAC procedures that can be life-threatening particularly in multiply comorbid, frail, patients. Frailty increases with age. Healing goes in the opposite direction; the speed of endothelialization reduces with age.

Conceptually we seem to be tying ourselves in knots by ring-fencing LAAC for those patients who are now too frail to take OAC safely. Such patients may be unable to scar the device quickly/completely and may have a lifespan dictated by their comorbidities. As such, they may be more vulnerable to the complications that younger, fitter, patients may survive. Equally they may simply not live long enough for the potential benefits of the procedure to accrue.

This seems a bizarre position to take. The natural history of AF is not controversial. As such there would seem to be a large window of opportunity to close/excise the LAA much earlier in the disease process before comorbidities of later life accrue which both limit the use of OAC (used to treat DRT) or compound adverse clinical events such as cardiac perforation. Repositioning the LAAC discussion to early after an AF diagnosis, rather than deferring it to the time that the patient fails first-line therapy with a life-threatening bleed or stroke has considerable merit and should be subject to a dedicated clinical trial.

The relevant clinical population would probably be in their early sixties before transition into the inevitable high-risk CHA$_2$DS$_2$-VASc bracket that accompanies aging. Clearly, the follow-up for such a study would be expected to be longer than we have seen in LAAC trials to date as the event rate to some extent requires the accumulation of risk. This situation is perhaps akin to the PFOc trials that followed patients for at least 5 years.[29–31] Interestingly, the subgroup analysis of the LAAOSIII study[4] (which recruited patients with CHA$_2$DS$_2$-VASc 2+) seems to show more utility of LAA excision (by any surgical method) for those patients with a CHA$_2$DS$_2$-VASc 2 to 4 (HR with 95% CI of 0.57 (0.40–0.82)) rather than the 5+ group (0.77 (0.56–1.06)) that makes a significant proportion of this trial cohort (the average CHA$_2$DS$_2$-VASc was 4.2). This is perhaps not surprising as the CHA$_2$DS$_2$-VASc score itself is dominated by atherosclerotic risk factors which elevate stroke risk irrespective of the presence of atrial fibrillation.[32] At a time most LAAC trials are heading toward higher risk cohorts (average CHA$_2$DS$_2$-VASc >4) this observation makes an important point about looking toward the other end of the scale.

In summary, if LAAC is useful at preventing stroke, early implantation should (1) decrease procedure risk, (2) facilitate early/complete endothelialization, (3) maximize medical options to treat DRT if it happens, and (4) maximizing the life years of therapy diluting the cost across decades of life rather than years.

It will not have escaped the reader's attention that there is very little consolation to be gained by the patient transitioning from a low (<2) into a high CHA$_2$DS$_2$-VASc (2+) bracket, and OAC eligibility, because of an index stroke. It may be wishful thinking to imagine that a mechanical device in the left atrium could change this, but we know already that the safety profile of OAC (specifically major bleeding) precludes net benefit of early OAC use for the large number of patients who fall into the lowest stroke risk categories. Hence there is a clear rationale for reassessing which patients may have the best outcomes from LAAC—the elderly high risk, or the younger apparently low risk. Moving the goalposts to the lower age range may have to wait for procedure safety to be improved (ie, better than OAC bleeding rates) before someone will be brave enough to sponsor this kind of study. But it should be done.

*In 5 years we will have a trial of LAAC for low-risk young patients, in less than 10 years we will have an answer. This will shift practice to lower risk patients who have yet to demonstrate bleeding risk.*

## PREDICTION 6: CHANGES IN DEVICE CONCEPT

The LAA has a variable morphology with an asymmetric, typically oval, orifice.[33] All intracardiac devices are symmetric. To deliver closure, in simple terms, all the current devices stretch the heart around the device. Even then what is claimed as closure is really the absence of a leak <5 mm—not anatomically complete closure which seems to hover around the 50% to 75% mark depending on what device is used,[9] and what method is used to investigate closure.[34] Defining closure in these terms may be too lax as cerebral vessels are 2–3 mm in diameter.[35] Hence a leak <5 mm will not prevent a clot escaping which could block a cerebral artery and cause a large stroke.

Stretching the heart incompletely around a device is not an ideal situation whereby underlying consequences of atrial fibrillation render the atrial tissue mechanically weak—"like wet blotting paper" in the words of one of our favorite surgeons. Furthermore, all the devices in current use have some sort of barb, hook, or anchor to keep it in the appendage. Yet we know the LAA is a thin-walled structure[36] and at risk of perforation from the anchors which can even extend into adjacent vascular structures.[37–42] If the stubborn pericardial effusion rate during LAAC of 1% is due to small perforations of the LAA, do we need to think of a completely different device concept that does not traumatize the LAA as much? In the next 10 years, after we know this is a procedure worth doing, we might see a completely disruptive approach to this problem.

By now we can imagine that the major device manufacturers have explored ways to inject various forms of intravascular Polyfilla into the LAA in a variety of 3D printed or animal models. The risk of embolization of such an approach may be considerable, particularly if the LAA volume expands and contracts over the course of the day which would be the natural assumption from the invasive pressure monitoring devices, but perhaps someone will come up with a clever way to fill and seal the appendage rather than block it.

The advantages would be multiple. There would be unlimited flexibility for patient anatomy, indeed, the various cracks and crevices in the LAA would be needed to anchor these devices making it better for more complex anatomy. The delivery system could be as small as the catheters used to opacify the appendage with contrast, simplifying the procedure enormously. Trauma, recapturing, hooks and perforations would be consigned to history.

How likely is this? Not very, but it would be a holy grail if it could be delivered.

## PREDICTION 7: CHANGES IN PROCEDURE—SAFETY

Although the procedure complication rates associated with LAAC are well cataloged, and encouragingly diminishing with increased operator/institutional experience[43] the fact remains that for a procedure that impacts the probabilistic chance of a future event—that is not an immediate threat—the major complication rate for this procedure needs to be as close to zero as it can be. As such improving safety must be a priority for the field.

This is likely to be a multi-pronged effort of marginal gains in many areas. Improving patient selection to reduce the "cohort C" type outcomes seen in TAVI will be married with improved preprocedure imaging to trim down both the 1% to 2% major complication and also the 1% to 2% procedure failure rates that expose patients to attempted—but ultimately unsuccessful closure attempts.

Physician training and a clearer understanding of both the "learning curve," and procedure volume to maintain an optimal service will improve. It seems churlish to assume that with the great anatomic complexity seen in the human LAA[33] and the high-stakes imposed by the typical patient frailty that acceptable numbers would be less than those recommended for simpler double-disc occluder procedures in the atrial mass—for example, ASD or PFO.[44,45] In that context the current proctoring industry standards of 5 to 10 cases seem insufficient and will likely need to increase in one form or another (eg, virtually[46]) particularly for the first device adopted by an operator/institution. The impact of volume is not just a catheter laboratory phenomenon; it has institutional impacts which improve case selection and postprocedure care which all contribute to safety metrics. It would seem logical to grow services from single leads working as part of a dedicated heart–brain team, taking on additional devices or operators only when volumes cross training or credentialing thresholds.

Improvements in aspects of the procedure which confer definite risk will occur. Transeptal puncture is an obvious example with systems now developed to stabilize the needle (eg TSP crossover[47]), replace the mechanical action of puncture with radiofrequency (eg Baylis NRG[48]), and reduce the need for wire exchanges (eg Versacross[49]) all likely to reduce one of the sources of cardiac perforation. With increased procedure familiarity, and supported by detailed upfront CT imaging,[50] adoption of intracardiac echo[51] to avoid the need for general anesthesia will improve safety in a cohort that is often a good candidate for LAAC but a poor candidate for GA. Improvements in the devices and their delivery systems will reduce the average number of devices, and deployments, to PFOC-like numbers of almost one.

Steerable sheath technology seems to offer clear advantages to align the device with the body of the appendage independently of the position of the transeptal puncture—which as a result could become increasingly central (and hence safe) rather than inferior (and posterior). As the distal end of these sheaths will have to retain angulation as the device is advanced, they will be more rigid (and thicker) than the nonsteerable equivalents. To not straighten, the sheath must be stiffer than the device/cable being pushed through it. Larger, stiffer, delivery systems could potentially cause as many problems as they fix. Something to help the operator avoid catheter perforation could be useful. Hence there may be considerable advantages incorporating pressure sensors required for contact force mapping found in some ablation catheters into LAAC delivery systems as it is often difficult to visualize the end of the catheter and determine its proximity to the LAA wall with current 2D imaging due to the curvature of the LAA.

The devices themselves will probably iterate to softer versions with less radial and longitudinal strength. The anchor mechanism may get smaller—perhaps with a general trend trading size for number (ie, more smaller anchors). Occasionally, in spite of all the preclinical work that goes into the process of device development—mistakes will occur and some device iterations will develop frame fractures, or not grip, and embolize as a result. This will require trips back to the drawing board, and the cath lab for industry and the patient, respectively.

*The procedure will continue to get safer as a result of marginal gains at nearly every stage.*

## PREDICTION 8: CHANGES IN PROCEDURE - EFFICACY

Efficacy is a composite of clinical benefits accrued after procedural harms are accounted for. Therefore, all the measures to improve safety contribute to efficacy. Can efficacy be further improved? Almost certainly. It is now clear that DRT is associated with some postprocedure stroke. Risk factors for DRT are now known for the implant[17] and the patient[52] and with increased planning it may either be possible to screen out patients likely to develop DRT or choose implantation strategies that make this less likely.[33,50] Certainly, accepting suboptimal, but stable, device outcomes should become a thing of the past as, much like TAVI, it becomes clearer whereby the boundaries between optimal and suboptimal outcomes lay.

The risk of DRT seems to be more clinically impactful in the first 12 months.[19] For patients treated with the intention to reduce stroke risk a more intensive early pharmacotherapy may become routine, particularly as studies like the AMULET IDE trial report that bleeding differences do not materialize within the Watchman arm (early OAC for 45d) compared with the Amulet arm (APT only).[9]

Although there is no contemporary data to show that residual leaks matter, complete closure will become an increasing focus for device development. Whether this translates to a clinical benefit is speculative but in simple terms patients, and their referring teams, want/expect appendage closure—not partial coverage. There are really no examples in contemporary cardiology whereby an incomplete result is not ultimately shown to be inferior to a complete result (eg, paravalve leak post-TAVI, incomplete coronary stent expansion, incomplete ablation lines, and so forth). If LAAC devices routinely achieve complete closure one of the reasons for postprocedure follow-up will be eliminated. If all patients have an intensified 1y medical prophylaxis for DRT this will remove the other indication to screen for DRT. This will have solidified in less than 10 years.

Tolerating leak thresholds larger than the cerebral vessels we are trying to protect should not be acceptable. Just as pacing rates post-TAVI give an indication of service quality, residual leaks may become quality metrics for LAAC services. This will probably become a feature in less than 5 years—particularly as centers begin to compete for eligible patients within treatment networks.

Efficacy may also improve if stroke attribution to cardiac embolism versus alternative mechanisms is enabled by better radiological imaging of the brain or circulating biomarkers. LAAC cannot reasonably be expected to prevent all strokes—only those potentially attributable to the LAA, but currently all stroke recurrence is equivalent. This muddies the water of exactly what LAAc is achieving in a complex jigsaw puzzle of stroke before/after device closure whereby multiple mechanisms coexist.

Equally if anatomic and physiologic factors of the left atrium (and the LAA) derived from cardiac imaging become a feature of stroke risk estimation, efficacy may be improved by targeting LAAC to those with the features more likely to benefit from a mechanical solution in the heart. Similarly, if AF-specific biomarkers of thrombogenicity were identified, the cohort of patients who need systemic anticoagulation (and who would be high risk for DRT) could be streamlined to OAC in preference to LAAc. The most bankable of these seems to be artificial intelligence lead efforts utilizing heart and brain imaging which seem to have 5 to 10y timelines for clinical translation.

*Efficacy of LAAC will improve through patient screening, device design, increased understanding of optimal deployment, optimized peri-procedure medication, and imaging-based stroke classification.*

## PREDICTION 9: CHANGES IN PATIENT INDICATION—BLEEDING RISK REDUCTION OR STROKE PREVENTION?

At times LAAC aspires to offer both reductions in ischemic stroke, and bleeding, a position that may be neither realistic nor obtainable. Trying to hold this moral high ground with data that doesn't exactly back the view at the present time harms the credibility of the field in the court of public opinion. OAC reduces ischemic stroke at the expense of bleeding. Is it a failure to position LAAC as the other side of that coin (reduced bleeding and hemorrhagic stroke, but with less impact on ischemic stroke)? After all, this is what the current data demonstrates,[53] and a significant number of patients with AF run a mile from the prospect of a blood thinner[54] in the short or medium term. This may only be a temporary staging post, but isn't this where we are until other trials emerge?

We focus heavily on $CHA_2DS_2$-VASc and the impact on stroke reduction, but for patients who have had a major bleed—and know what that means—the absence of bleeding (and the fear of bleeding) may be just as laudable as any contribution toward stroke prevention. Indeed, we typically see in the European LAAC registries[15,55,56] the dominant reason for LAAC is a major bleed (70% in the Amulet registry, 60% in EWOLUTION) rather than prior stroke (27% in the Amulet registry, 40% in EWOLUTION). Are we looking at a glass half empty, when really the glass is half full?

In this regard do we need to work out which high-risk bleeding patients are the best to treat? Presently this is not done well. A patient who has a major bleed without exposure to OAC may have less to gain from LAAC than a patient who plausibly bleeds because of the OAC they may subsequently be able to avoid. This distinction is important and amplified by the dilemma of treating DRT, which is more complex in the first example than the second.

What about those who are yet to have a major bleed? The risk predictors are about as good for bleeding as they are for stroke. Is there a reason to privilege one scoring system more than the other? Within the spectrum of patients naïve to OAC, there are bound to be a significant number in whom bleeding risk predominates, for whom the best treatment option may well be LAAC, rather than nothing, or a trial of OAC to precipitate a bleed that facilitates decision making.

*It may transpire, in a ~5y timeframe, that LAAC becomes less a stroke prevention procedure, and more a way to limit bleeding risk as improved ways to determine the net benefit patients may derive from all options available emerge.*

## PREDICTION 10: THE SPECIAL CASE OF LAAC IN PATIENTS WITH PRIOR INTRACEREBRAL HEMORRHAGE

Patients with prior intracerebral hemorrhage (ICH) and AF represent an important group of patients for whom LAAC is sometimes considered. The major DOAC trials have clearly shown the superiority of DOACs over vitamin K antagonists regarding hemorrhagic stroke risk,[57] with around half the odds of hemorrhagic stroke in patients taking DOACs. Even if hemorrhagic stroke is less likely on DOACs, ICHs on DOACs are still often catastrophic, life-threatening events and the risk of these occurring is a significant cause of anxiety for clinicians resuming or starting anticoagulation in such patients.[58] Although specific reversal agents are now available, considerable damage is often done before a reversal can be administered. On the other side of the coin, these patients are at high risk of ischemic stroke and major vascular events, with an incidence of 15.5 per 100 patient-years compared with 3.3 per 100 patient-years for recurrent ICH in a combined analysis of pooled, population-based, ICH cohorts,[59] so leaving these patients without anticoagulation leaves them exposed to an even higher risk of ischemic complications.

Recent small clinical trials randomizing these patients to avoid or start an anticoagulant suggest that starting anticoagulation might be superior to avoiding anticoagulation for preventing symptomatic major vascular events.[60] Although numbers were small in the SoSTART pilot trial, twice the number of recurrent ICHs were seen in the anticoagulated group and of these ICHs, 7 out of 8 were fatal, compared with no deaths in the 4 recurrent ICHs in the avoid group. Ongoing trials addressing the same question should provide definitive answers, but if we continue to see an increase in fatal recurrent ICH there will remain an unmet need for a treatment that avoids the potential harm of anticoagulation while providing the same benefits. There is also evidence that the profile of ICH is changing, with improved management of hypertension and an increasingly aged population leading to more ICH in patients with cerebral amyloid angiopathy[61] and less with hypertension. Bleeding risk is partly driven by etiology, being higher with cerebral amyloid angiopathy and lower with hypertensive microangiopathy,[62] so it may be that the harm done by anticoagulation increases as cerebral amyloid angiopathy becomes more prevalent in patients with AF. On the face of it, LAAC offers a solution to this, providing protection from systemic embolism without increasing the risk of recurrent ICH.

Based on results so far, it seems likely that starting an anticoagulant will be shown to be superior to avoiding one in patients with AF and prior ICH in a pooled analysis of the ongoing trials addressing this question in a combined cohort of over 3000 patients. Alongside this, ongoing trials are beginning to explore the option of LAAC, including the STROKECLOSE trial (NCT02830152), aiming to recruit 750 patients with a prior ICH who will be randomized to either LAAC or best medical therapy, at the clinician's discretion, which may include no antithrombotic or antiplatelets alone. This poses the problem of a heterogenous control arm but will begin to provide high-quality data comparing LAAC with DOAC treatment in this population. It is unlikely that this will be sufficient to answer the question and head-to-head trials of LAAC versus DOACs in patients with AF and prior ICH are likely to then follow. As the LAAC procedure improves while we wait to get to these trials, the chances of LAAC being shown superior to DOACs will gradually be increasing. Hopefully, LAAC will fulfill this ambition, meaning we no longer must accept a higher risk of catastrophic, recurrent ICH in our patients restarted on DOACs after their first ICH.

## SUMMARY

The commercial and clinical potential of a mechanical one-off solution to a common problem like the embolic complications of atrial fibrillation cannot be underestimated. Like the early experience with the transcatheter aortic valves, most of the early experience has been gained in high-risk patient groups with no other options— patients with LAAC too frail to take OAC. A randomized high-quality trial versus DOAC with a clear superiority outcome is likely to be needed to change international guidelines; but this may only be realized after significant iterations in patient evaluation, device development, and procedure execution are brought about. This is problematic because the DOAC patent expiry dates run along similar timelines and cost-effectiveness arguments for LAAC benefit from higher DOAC costs. Incorporating additional capabilities within LAA occluders could potentially broaden their acceptability to payers if they deliver additional health-economic benefits in heart failure. Predicting the future is hazardous, the value of the personal opinions expressed in this piece may go down, as well as up.

## CLINICS CARE POINTS

- Trials are underway evaluating existing LAA closure devices to direct oral anticoagulants
- The principle advantage of extracardiac LAA closure is the absence of intracardiac material and additional factors related to structural and electrical impacts not seen with intracardiac devices.
- The opportunity to incorporate hemodynamic assessment capabilities into LAAC devices may strengthen clinical utility and health economic arguments for intracardiac LAA closure.
- Further evolution of LAAC is likely to accelerate in the near future.

## REFERENCES

1. @pknoepfler twitter. Available at: https://twitter.com/pknoepfler/status/1349024982442143747?s=19. Accessed December 1, 2021.

2. Hellerstein HK, Sinaiko E, Dolgin M. Amputation of the canine atrial appendages. Proc Soc Exp Biol Med 1947;66(2):337.

3. Madden JL. Resection of the left auricular appendix; a prophylaxis for recurrent arterial emboli. J Am Med Assoc 1949;140(9):769–72.

4. Whitlock RP, Belley-Cote EP, Paparella D, et al. Left atrial appendage occlusion during cardiac surgery to prevent stroke. N Engl J Med 2021;384(22):2081–91. https://doi.org/10.1056/NEJMoa2101897.

5. Sievert H, Lesh MD, Trepels T, et al. Percutaneous left atrial appendage transcatheter occlusion to prevent stroke in high-risk patients with atrial fibrillation: early clinical experience. Circulation 2002;105(16):1887–9. https://doi.org/10.1161/01.CIR.0000015698.54752.6D.

6. Meier B, Palacios I, Windecker S, et al. Transcatheter left atrial appendage occlusion with Amplatzer devices to obviate anticoagulation in patients with atrial fibrillation. Catheter Cardiovasc Interv 2003;60(3):417–22.

7. Holmes DR, Reddy VY, Turi ZG, et al. Percutaneous closure of the left atrial appendage versus warfarin therapy for prevention of stroke in patients with atrial fibrillation: a randomised noninferiority trial. Lancet 2009;374:534–42. https://doi.org/10.1016/S0140-6736(09)61343-X.

8. Holmes DR Jr, Kar S, Price MJ, et al. Prospective randomized evaluation of the watchman left atrial appendage closure device in patients with atrial fibrillation versus long-term warfarin therapy: the PREVAIL trial. J Am Coll Cardiol 2014;64(1):1–12. https://doi.org/10.1016/j.jacc.2014.04.029. Erratum in: J Am Coll Cardiol. 2014 Sep 16;64(11):1186.

9. Lakkireddy D, Thaler D, Ellis CR, et al. AMPLATZER™ AMULET™ left atrial appendage Occluder versus watchman™ device for stroke prophylaxis (amulet ide): a randomized controlled trial. Circulation 2021. https://doi.org/10.1161/CIRCULATIONAHA.121.057063.

10. Kar S, Doshi SK, Sadhu A, et al, PINNACLE FLX Investigators. Primary outcome evaluation of a next-generation left atrial appendage closure device: results from the PINNACLE FLX trial. Circulation 2021;143(18):1754–62. https://doi.org/10.1161/CIRCULATIONAHA.120.050117.

11. Price MJ, Saw J. Transcatheter left atrial appendage occlusion in the DOAC era. J Am Coll Cardiol 2020;75(25):3136–9. https://doi.org/10.1016/j.jacc.2020.05.019.

12. Leon MB, Smith CR, Mack M, et al, PARTNER Trial Investigators. Transcatheter aortic-valve implantation for aortic stenosis in patients who cannot undergo surgery. N Engl J Med 2010;363(17):1597–607. https://doi.org/10.1056/NEJMoa1008232.

13. Sievert K, Asmarats L, Arzamendi D. LAAO the strengths and weaknesses of the lobe only occluder concept in theory and in practice. Interv Cardiol Clin, in press.

14. Wong I, Tzikas A, Søndergaard L, et al. The strengths and weaknesses of the LAA covering disc occluders – conceptually and in practice. Interv Cardiol Clin, in press.

15. Ledwoch J, Franke J, Akin I, et al. WATCHMAN versus ACP or Amulet devices for left atrial appendage occlusion: a sub-analysis of the multicentre LAARGE registry. Eurointervention 2020;16(11):e942–9. https://doi.org/10.4244/EIJ-D-19-01027.

16. Saw J, Nielsen-Kudsk JE, Bergmann M, et al. Rationale and choice of antithrombotic therapy following left atrial appendage closure. JACC Cardiovasc Interv 2019;12(11):1067–76. https://doi.org/10.1016/j.jcin.2018.11.001.

17. Aminian A, Schmidt B, Mazzone P, et al. Incidence, characterization, and clinical impact of device-related thrombus following left atrial appendage occlusion in the prospective global AMPLATZER amulet observational study. JACC Cardiovasc Interv 2019;12(11):1003–14. https://doi.org/10.1016/j.jcin.2019.02.003.

18. Mill J, Olivares AL, Arzamendi D, et al. Impact of flow dynamics on device-related thrombosis after left atrial appendage occlusion. Can J Cardiol

2020;36(6):968.e13–4. https://doi.org/10.1016/j.cjca.2019.12.036.

19. Dukkipati SR, Kar S, Holmes DR, et al. Device-related thrombus after left atrial appendage closure: incidence, predictors, and outcomes. Circulation 2018;138(9):874–85. https://doi.org/10.1161/CIRCULATIONAHA.118.035090.

20. Alkhouli M, Busu T, Shah K, et al. Incidence and clinical impact of device-related thrombus following percutaneous left atrial appendage occlusion: a meta-analysis. JACC Clin Electrophysiol 2018;4(12):1629–37. https://doi.org/10.1016/j.jacep.2018.09.007.

21. Lee RJ, Hanke T. The strengths and weaknesses of LAA ligation or exclusion (LARIAT, ATRIA-CLIP, Surgical suture). Interv Cardiol Clin, in press.

22. Abraham WT, Adamson PB, Bourge RC, et al, CHAMPION Trial Study Group. Wireless pulmonary artery haemodynamic monitoring in chronic heart failure: a randomised controlled trial. Lancet 2011;377(9766):658–66. https://doi.org/10.1016/S0140-6736(11)60101-3. Erratum in: Lancet. 2012 Feb 4;379(9814):412.

23. Sievert H, Di Mario C, Perl L, et al. VECTOR-HF: The first human experience with the V-LAP, a wireless left atrial pressure monitoring system for patients with heart failure. Eur Heart J 2019;40(Supplement_1). ehz745.0898.

24. Taylor JK, Ndiaye H, Daniels M, et al. Triage-HF Plus investigators. Lockdown, slow down: impact of the COVID-19 pandemic on physical activity-an observational study. Open Heart 2021;8(1):e001600. https://doi.org/10.1136/openhrt-2021-001600.

25. Marlevi D, Edelman ER. Vascular lesion-specific drug delivery systems: JACC state-of-the-art review. J Am Coll Cardiol 2021;77(19):2413–31. https://doi.org/10.1016/j.jacc.2021.03.307.

26. Asmarats L, Cruz-González I, Nombela-Franco L, et al. Recurrence of device-related thrombus after percutaneous left atrial appendage closure. Circulation 2019;140(17):1441–3. https://doi.org/10.1161/CIRCULATIONAHA.119.040860.

27. Wijffels MC, Kirchhof CJ, Dorland R, et al. Atrial fibrillation begets atrial fibrillation. A study in awake chronically instrumented goats. Circulation 1995;92(7):1954–68. https://doi.org/10.1161/01.cir.92.7.1954.

28. Abushouk AI, Ali AA, Mohamed AA, et al. Rhythm versus rate control for atrial fibrillation: a meta-analysis of randomized controlled trials. Biomed Pharmacol J 2018;11(2):609–20.

29. Mas JL, Derumeaux G, Guillon B, et al, CLOSE Investigators. Patent foramen ovale closure or anticoagulation vs. antiplatelets after stroke. N Engl J Med 2017;377(11):1011–21. https://doi.org/10.1056/NEJMoa1705915.

30. Saver JL, Carroll JD, Thaler DE, et al, RESPECT Investigators. Long-term outcomes of patent foramen ovale closure or medical therapy after stroke. N Engl J Med 2017;377(11):1022–32. https://doi.org/10.1056/NEJMoa1610057.

31. Søndergaard L, Kasner SE, Rhodes JF, et al, Gore REDUCE Clinical Study Investigators. Patent foramen ovale closure or antiplatelet therapy for cryptogenic stroke. N Engl J Med 2017;377(11):1033–42. https://doi.org/10.1056/NEJMoa1707404. Erratum in: N Engl J Med. 2020 Mar 5;382(10):978.

32. Siddiqi TJ, Usman MS, Shahid I, et al. Utility of the CHA2DS2-VASc score for predicting ischaemic stroke in patients with or without atrial fibrillation: a systematic review and meta-analysis. Eur J Prev Cardiol 2021;zwab018. https://doi.org/10.1093/eurjpc/zwab018.

33. Cresti A, Toscana S, Camara O. Left atrial thrombus – are all atria and appendages equal? Interv Cardiol Clin, in press.

34. Nestelberger T, Alfadhel M, McAlister, C, et al. Follow up imaging after left atrial appendage occlusion – something or nothing, and for how long? Interv Cardiol Clin, in press.

35. Reina-De La Torre F, Rodriguez-Baeza A, Sahuquillo-Barris J. Morphological characteristics and distribution pattern of the arterial vessels in human cerebral cortex: a scanning electron microscope study. Anat Rec 1998;251(1):87–96. https://doi.org/10.1002/(SICI)1097-0185(199805)251:1<87::AID-AR14>3.0.CO;2-7.

36. Park JW, Bethencourt A, Sievert H, et al. Left atrial appendage closure with Amplatzer cardiac plug in atrial fibrillation: initial European experience. Catheter Cardiovasc Interv 2011;77(5):700–6. https://doi.org/10.1002/ccd.22764. Erratum in: Catheter Cardiovasc Interv. 2014 Nov 15;84(6):1028. Lopez-Minquez, Jose Ramon [corrected to Lopez-Minguez, Jose Ramon].

37. Zwirner J, Bayer R, Hädrich C, et al. Pulmonary artery perforation and coronary air embolism-two fatal outcomes in percutaneous left atrial appendage occlusion. Int J Leg Med 2017;131(1):191–7.

38. Hanazawa K, Brunelli M, Saenger J, et al. Close proximity between pulmonary artery and left atrial appendage leading to perforation of the artery, tamponade and death after appendage closure using cardiac plug device. Int J Cardiol 2014;175(2):e35–6.

39. Sepahpour A, Ng MK, Storey P, et al. Death from pulmonary artery erosion complicating implantation of percutaneous left atrial appendage occlusion device. Heart Rhythm 2013;10(12):1810–1.

40. Halkin A, Cohen C, Rosso R, et al. Left atrial appendage and pulmonary artery anatomic relationship by cardiac-gated computed tomography:

implications for late pulmonary artery perforation by left atrial appendage closure devices. Heart Rhythm 2016;13(10):2064–9.

41. Lu C, Zeng J, Meng Q, et al. Pulmonary artery perforation caused by a left atrial appendage closure device. Catheter Cardiovasc Interv 2019. https://doi.org/10.1002/ccd.28541.

42. Pracoń R, De Backer O, Konka M, et al. Imaging risk features for device related pulmonary artery injury after left atrial appendage closure with Amplatzer™ Amulet™ device. Catheter Cardiovasc Interv 2020. https://doi.org/10.1002/ccd.29393.

43. Nazir S, Ahuja KR, Kolte D, et al. Association of hospital procedural volume with outcomes of percutaneous left atrial appendage occlusion. JACC Cardiovasc Interv 2021;14(5):554–61. https://doi.org/10.1016/j.jcin.2020.11.029.

44. Marmagkiolis K, Hakeem A, Cilingiroglu M, et al. The society for cardiovascular angiography and interventions structural heart disease early career task force survey results: endorsed by the society for cardiovascular angiography and interventions. Catheter Cardiovasc Interv 2012;80(4):706–11. https://doi.org/10.1002/ccd.24535.

45. Armsby L, Beekman RH 3rd, Benson L, et al. SCAI expert consensus statement for advanced training programs in pediatric and congenital interventional cardiac catheterization. Catheter Cardiovasc Interv 2014;84(5):779–84. https://doi.org/10.1002/ccd.25550.

46. Goel SS, Greenbaum AB, Patel A, et al. Role of teleproctoring in challenging and innovative structural interventions amid the COVID-19 pandemic and beyond. JACC Cardiovasc Interv 2020;13(16):1945–8. https://doi.org/10.1016/j.jcin.2020.04.013.

47. Russo G, Taramasso M, Maisano F. Transseptal puncture: a step-by-step procedural guide. Card Interventions Today 2019;13:22–6.

48. Sherman W, Lee P, Hartley A, et al. Transatrial septal catheterization using a new radiofrequency probe. Catheter Cardiovasc Interv 2005;66:14–7.

49. Sayah N, Simon F, Garceau P, et al. Initial clinical experience with VersaCross transseptal system for transcatheter mitral valve repair. Catheter Cardiovasc Interv 2021;97(6):1230–4. https://doi.org/10.1002/ccd.29365.

50. Devgun J, De Potter T, Fabbricatore D, et al. Pre-Cath Lab Planning for Left Atrial Appendage Occlusion – Optional or Essential? Interv Cardiol Clin, in press.

51. Alkhouli M, Nielsen-Kudsk JE. The case for intracardiac echo to Guide left atrial appendage closure. Interv Cardiol Clin, in press.

52. Simard T, Jung RG, Lehenbauer K, et al. Predictors of device-related thrombus following percutaneous left atrial appendage occlusion. J Am Coll Cardiol 2021;78(4):297–313. https://doi.org/10.1016/j.jacc.2021.04.098.

53. Saraf K, Morris, GM. Left Atrial Appendage Closure: what the evidence does and does not reveal – a view from the outside. Interv Cardiol Clin, in press.

54. Ding WY, Lip GYH, Gupta D. Left atrial appendage occlusion – a choice or a last resort? How to approach the patient. Interv Cardiol Clin, in press.

55. Boersma LV, Schmidt B, Betts TR, et al. EWOLUTION investigators. Implant success and safety of left atrial appendage closure with the WATCHMAN device: peri-procedural outcomes from the EWOLUTION registry. Eur Heart J 2016; 37(31):2465–74. https://doi.org/10.1093/eurheartj/ehv730.

56. Hildick-Smith D, Landmesser U, Camm AJ, et al. Left atrial appendage occlusion with the Amplatzer™ Amulet™ device: full results of the prospective global observational study. Eur Heart J 2020;41(30):2894–901. https://doi.org/10.1093/eurheartj/ehaa169.

57. Makam RCP, Hoaglin DC, McManus DD, et al. Efficacy and safety of direct oral anticoagulants approved for cardiovascular indications: Systematic review and meta-analysis. PLoS One 2018;13(5): e0197583. https://doi.org/10.1371/journal.pone.0197583.

58. Wilson D, Seiffge DJ, Traenka C, et al. Outcome of intracerebral hemorrhage associated with different oral anticoagulants. Neurology 2017;88(18):1693–700. https://doi.org/10.1212/WNL.0000000000003886. Erratum in: Neurology. 2018 Jun 5;90(23):1084.

59. Li L, Poon MTC, Samarasekera NE, et al. Risks of recurrent stroke and all serious vascular events after spontaneous intracerebral haemorrhage: pooled analyses of two population-based studies. Lancet Neurol 2021;20(6):437–47. https://doi.org/10.1016/S1474-4422(21)00075-2. Erratum in: Lancet Neurol. 2021 Jun 9.

60. SoSTART Collaboration. Effects of oral anticoagulation for atrial fibrillation after spontaneous intracranial haemorrhage in the UK: a randomised, open-label, assessor-masked, pilot-phase, non-inferiority trial. Lancet Neurol 2021. https://doi.org/10.1016/S1474-4422(21)00264-7.

61. Béjot Y, Cordonnier C, Durier J, et al. Intracerebral haemorrhage profiles are changing: results from the Dijon population-based study. Brain 2013; 136(Pt 2):658–64. https://doi.org/10.1093/brain/aws349.

62. Pinho J, Araújo JM, Costa AS, et al. Intracerebral hemorrhage recurrence in patients with and without cerebral amyloid angiopathy. Cerebrovasc Dis Extra 2021;11(1):15–21. https://doi.org/10.1159/000513503.

# Moving?

## Make sure your subscription moves with you!

To notify us of your new address, find your **Clinics Account Number** (located on your mailing label above your name), and contact customer service at:

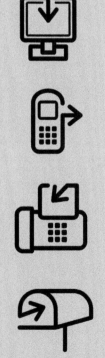

**Email: journalscustomerservice-usa@elsevier.com**

**800-654-2452** (subscribers in the U.S. & Canada)
**314-447-8871** (subscribers outside of the U.S. & Canada)

**Fax number: 314-447-8029**

**Elsevier Health Sciences Division
Subscription Customer Service
3251 Riverport Lane
Maryland Heights, MO 63043**

*To ensure uninterrupted delivery of your subscription, please notify us at least 4 weeks in advance of move.

ELSEVIER

Printed and bound by CPI Group (UK) Ltd, Croydon, CR0 4YY

03/10/2024

01040367-0004